Essential Biochemistry and Genetics for Medicine

By Stefano Palazzo

TWIN SERPENTS LIMITED
OXFORD, UK

Published by Twin Serpents Limited 2010   ISBN 978–1–905524–14–3

ABOUT THE AUTHOR

Stefano Palazzo read pre-clinical and clinical Medicine at Somerville and Green Templeton Colleges at the University of Oxford, graduating in 2010. Whilst an undergraduate at Somerville he gained a distinguished academic record, being awarded a First Class degree and receiving the Gibbs Prize for one of the most outstanding examination performance in the Finals Examinations of 2007. He continued to excel in his clinical studies between 2008 and 2010. During this time he was appointed as a tutor in Biochemistry and Medical Genetics at Somerville, teaching medical undergraduates in the first year of their pre-clinical studies. His inspirational and very successful approach to teaching medical undergraduates provided the basis the material presented in this book.

Dr Matthew Wood, Fellow and Tutor in Medicine, Somerville College, Oxford

TABLE OF CONTENTS

CHAPTER 1

Protein Structure and Function

1.1 GENERAL PRINCIPLES OF BIOCHEMICAL STRUCTURES

Biological molecules rely on their macromolecular organisation and structure for their function. This applies to proteins, lipids and carbohydrates, as well as the larger structures that they form. Macromolecular organisation depends upon interactions at the level of the individual units, as well as between chains or complexes of two or more units.

Stereoisomerism
- Stereoisomers are molecules whose atomic structures are the same, but arrangement in space is different.
- Amino acids and some monosaccharides in particular exist as stereoisomers, often as enantiomers (non-superimposable mirror images of a molecule, arranged tetrahedrally around a chiral (almost always carbon) centre – classified as either L or D-forms).
- Important biologically since their interactions and function vary e.g. only L-form amino acids found in eukaryotic proteins, whereas D-forms found in bacterial cell walls and some antibiotics.

1.2 PROTEINS

1.2.1 General Principles
Proteins perform a number of important roles in biology, and come in various functional forms, for which they are specialised:

Structural – support (extracellular matrix proteins, keratin, fibroin), barrier and motility (cytoskeleton e.g. actin and myosin, bacterial flagellae) functions.

Enzymes – biological catalysts e.g. lactate dehydrogenase.

Transporters – translocatory proteins used to move substances across otherwise impermeable cells membranes (e.g. glucose transporter GLUT), within or between cells (e.g. haemoglobin) and transduce a signal (e.g. acetylcholine receptor).

Regulatory – control of activity of other proteins (e.g. allosteric inhibitors of enzymes) or interaction with non-protein structures (e.g. transcription factors binding to DNA).

1.2.2 Protein Composition and Structure

1.2.2.1 Amino Acids and the Peptide Bond
Amino acids are the 'building blocks' of proteins, with proteins from all species made from the same set of 20 *standard* amino acids, classified according to their functional side chains. The general structure is NH_2-CHR-COOH – i.e. central carbon atom (α-carbon atom) with adjacent primary amino and carboxylic acid groups.

Amino acids are normally zwitterionic (neutral at *body* pH) but their side groups can be classified:

Basic – amino groups on side chains positively charged at *neutral* pH (N.B. not body pH) e.g. arginine, lysine.

Acidic – carboxyl groups of side chains negatively charged (i.e. deprotonated) at neutral pH e.g. aspartic acid, glutamic acid.

Hydrophilic – basic and acidic amino acids (as outlined above) as well as histidines, which have polar, hydrophilic side-chains.

Hydrophobic – amino acids with hydrophobic (due to presence of aliphatic side chains or aromatic rings) functional groups. Includes glycine, proline and cysteine.

Structural – used to described proline, which is hydrophobic but, by virtue of its aliphatic side-chain bonded back onto the amino group, is conformationally rigid.

The peptide bond is a covalent bond linking the α-amino group of one amino acid to the α-carboxyl group of another to form a dipeptide. This has the characteristics of a partial double-bond and limits rotation around it (though free rotation does take place around the bonds either side of the peptide linkage). This has important implications for secondary structure since it defines the interactions that are able to take place in motifs such as α-helices and β-pleated sheets.

Formation of a peptide bond involves the release of water:

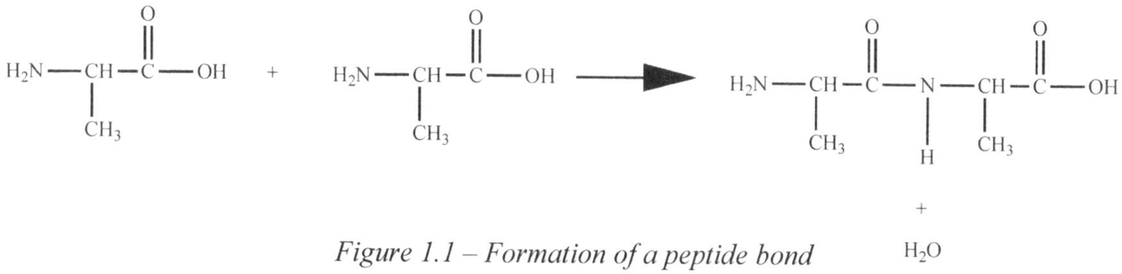

Figure 1.1 – Formation of a peptide bond H_2O

Apart from glycine, all amino acids have four different groups arranged tetrahedrally around a (chiral) carbon centre. This confers chirality, with two non-superimposable, mirror-image enantiomers of each amino acid existing (L and D forms). This has implications for the shape (and hence functions) of proteins, and thus when developing drugs a consideration of stereoisomerism is extremely important (e.g. penicillin, thalidomide – one form prevents morning sickness, one form is teratogenic).

1.2.2.2 Principles of Protein Structure
The three-dimensional conformation of a protein (beyond the peptide bonds between individual amino acids) is maintained by various covalent and non-covalent interactions:

Van der Waal's forces – non-covalent interaction between electrically neutral molecules due to electrostatic interactions between permanent and/or induced dipoles.

Hydrogen bonds – electrostatic interactions between a hydrogen atom covalently attached to an oxygen or nitrogen atom (causing it to be δ^+) and an acceptor atom (oxygen or nitrogen in biological systems) that bears a lone pair of electrons (making it δ^-). Stronger than van der Waal's forces, but significantly weaker than covalent bonds.

Hydrophobic forces – forces caused by the movement of hydrophobic groups (e.g. non-polar side chains of individual amino acids) on an amphipathic molecule in an attempt to avoid contact with water.

Ionic interactions – interaction between two ionic groups of opposite charge e.g. ammonium group of lysine and carboxyl group of aspartate to form a 'salt bridge'.

Disulphide bond – covalent bonds that form between two cysteine residues which are close together in a protein. Very strong forces, and therefore function to stabilise the 3D structure.

Polypeptide chains fold up to form a specific conformation in the protein, dependent on the amino acid sequence, which has four levels of organisation:

Primary
The number and sequence of amino acids in a polypeptide chain joined by covalent peptide linkages. Ultimately determined by the genetic code. Also includes the position of additional covalent bonds, mainly disulphide linkages.

Significance to protein sequencing techniques, as well as the effect of mutation on the subsequent secondary and tertiary structure e.g. cystic fibrosis caused by point mutation in the CFTR gene, leading to incorrect folding and faulty protein function.

Secondary
Describes the folding of regions of the polypeptide chain giving regular spatial arrangements. Stabilised by molecular interactions, particularly hydrogen bonds, van der Waal's forces and electro-static interactions.

There are a few common (and functionally important) secondary motifs:

α-HELICES
Rod-like structures, in which amino acids arrange themselves in a regular helical conformation. Possesses 3.6 amino acids per turn, and the side chains are arranged around the outside of the central helix.

Formed by hydrogen bonds between the oxygen in the C=O of the peptide bond, and the hydrogen in the N-H of the peptide bond four amino acids away. Certain amino acids are rarely found in α-helices, such as proline (lack of a hydrogen atom on its nitrogen preventing proper hydrogen bonding).

Found in the structural protein keratin (hair and nails) where two or more helices intertwine to form very stable structures.

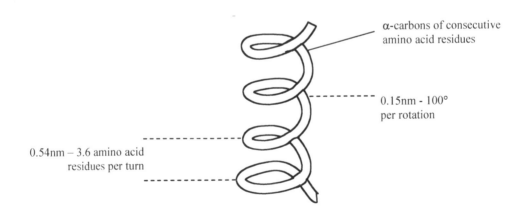

α-carbons of consecutive amino acid residues

0.15nm - 100° per rotation

0.54nm – 3.6 amino acid residues per turn

Figure 1.2 – Schematic diagram of an α-helix

12

Sheet formed by hydrogen bonds between the peptide bonds either in different polypeptide chains, or the same polypeptide chain folded back on itself – adjacent chains either parallel (run in same direction) or antiparallel (run in opposite direction i.e. C-N and N-C). Side chains protrude above and below the sheet, with planarity of the peptide bond resulting in the pleating.

When the sheet consists of chains from the same polypeptide sequence, the polypeptide sequence makes a tight hairpin turn (β-turn). Interactions between the stretches either side of the turn stabilise it, and allow reversal of the direction of the sequence.

Present in the protein fibroin (found in silk) where they give both strength and flexibility (ability to slide over each other).

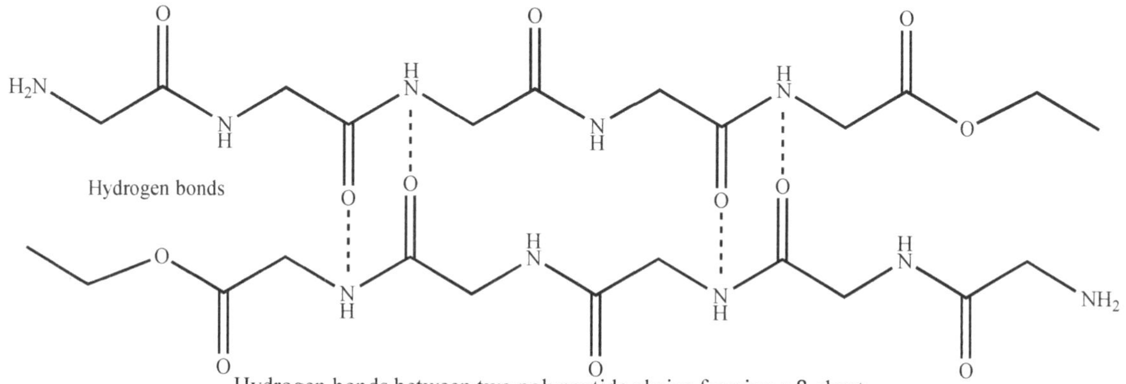

Hydrogen bonds

Hydrogen bonds between two polypeptide chains forming a β-sheet

Folding of a polypeptide chain into a β-turn

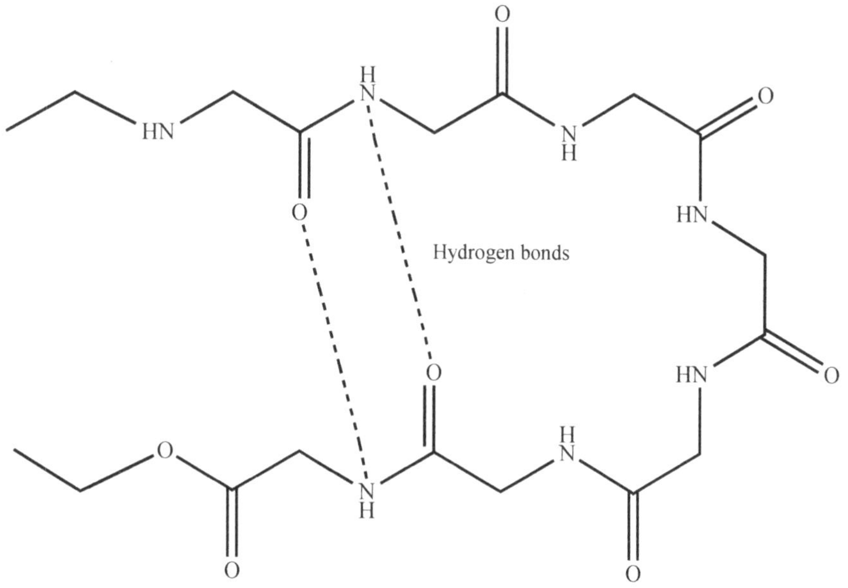

Hydrogen bonds

Figure 1.3 – Molecular structure of the β-pleated sheet and β-turn

13

LOOPS
Around 50% of the polypeptide chain of a typical globular protein is not contained within regular secondary structures. These regions are said to have a loop or coil conformation.

tertiary
Describes the conformation that arises due to spatial arrangement of amino acids that are both adjacent and far away in the linear sequence.

Tertiary structure arises due to thermodynamically driven folding of the polypeptide sequence. In globular proteins, such as myoglobin, the main driving force is the movement of hydrophobic amino acids/side chains away from an aqueous environment. Once folded into the correct conformation, the protein is stabilised by distant electrostatic interactions, hydrogen bonding and disulphide linkages.

Folding into a tertiary structure leads to the formation of both structural and functional domains – groups of motifs. This is particularly important to proteins such as enzymes, whose active site shapes, with catalytic and binding domains in the cleft, require specific tertiary arrangement to provide a suitable environment. Similarly, receptor proteins (e.g. LDL receptors – mutation leads to familial hypercholesterolemia due to incorrect tertiary structure) and transporters such as myoglobin (eight helices combine into extremely compact structure, whilst has haem prosthetic group localised in a hydrophobic crevice where conditions are perfect for function) rely on tertiary structure.

Quaternary
Quaternary structure describes the assembly of multiple protein chains (subunits) into a complete functional protein unit, stabilised by covalent or non-covalent interactions. May be either homo- or hetero-oligomeric, depending on whether the subunits are identical (homo-oligomeric) or different.

Good example is haemoglobin, which shows allosteric regulation. It consists of four subunits (two α, two β) and is able to bind four molecules of oxygen. Binding of oxygen to one subunit leads to a conformational change in the other subunits, increasing their affinity for subsequent oxygen molecules. This is known as cooperative behaviour, and results in the sigmoidal oxygen dissociation curve (in contrast to the non-cooperative binding of the single subunit of myoglobin).

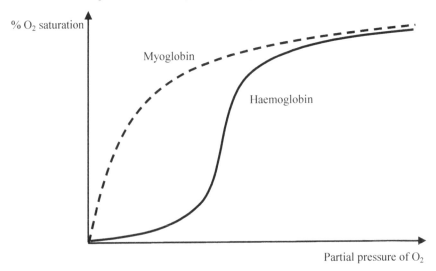

Figure 1.4 – Oxygen dissociation curves for myoglobin and haemoglobin

Sickle cell anaemia – change from glutamic acid to valine in the β-chain of haemoglobin alters hydrophobic interactions. This causes long haemoglobin fibres to aggregate and distort the shape of erythrocytes, resulting in their sickle appearance and blocked blood flow in narrow capillaries.

Other important proteins with multiple subunits include antibodies, formed by combination of various chains (variable and constant regions) facilitating their roles in immunity.

Multiprotein complexes
Complexes of various proteins can form, allowing interactions for more efficient function. For example, pyruvate dehydrogenase consists of the complex of various enzymes with close proximity leading to efficient and rapid catalysis without the loss of intermediates (substrate passed from enzyme E1 to E2 to E3).

1.2.3 STRUCTURAL PROTEINS – STRUCTURE AND FUNCTION

1.2.3.1 Collagen
Collagen is a family of structurally related proteins (classically 5 different types of collagen, with slightly different properties), and is the most abundant protein in mammals. The various forms act to anchor cells within organs as part of the extracellular matrix, and are also the major fibrous elements of skin, bones, tendons, ligaments, cartilage, blood vessels and teeth. The molecular structure is specialised for strength, particularly in tendons (type 1 collagen), which have extremely high tensile strength.

Primary structure – each polypeptide in collagen consists of repeating tripeptide sequence Gly-X-Y, where X is often proline and Y is often hydroxyproline.

Secondary structure – the polypeptide chains are around 1000 residues long and fold up into a unique and characteristic collagen helix (N.B. different to the α-helix).

Quaternary structure – three polypeptide chains wind around each other (slightly right hand twist) to form a triple-helical cable. The arrangement of the chains in this triple helix necessitates glycine every third residue since only the small side chain of this amino acid can fit in its centre. The chains are also staggered so the glycine of one chain, X of another and Y of another are all aligned. Extensive hydrogen bonds help to stabilise the helix, as do the hydroxyl groups of hydroxyproline and the inflexibility of proline and hydroxyproline. Formation of this helix (which occurs within fibroblasts) requires extension peptide sequences containing cysteine, which also prevent premature aggregation within the cell.

Multi-protein complex – the triple helices with extension peptides (called procollagen) are secreted from fibroblasts. Following this, the extension peptides are cleaved by extracellular peptidases resulting in tropocollagen, which aggregate together in a staggered head-to-tail arrangement in the collagen fibre. The strength and rigidity of collagen fibres is dependent upon covalent cross-links between and within tropocollagen molecules – often between lysine residues and its aldehyde derivative allysine (formation requires lysyl oxidase).

There are various clinical conditions involving collagen, both genetic and environment-related:
- Scurvy – vitamin C deficiency, resulting in failure of hydroxyproline (and hydroxylysine) synthesis since their synthase enzymes (proline hydroxylase, lysine hydroxylase) require the vitamin as a co-factor.

- Osteogenesis imperfecta – 'brittle bone disease' due to primary structure mutation, often a glycine substitution resulting in disruption of folding and triple helix formation. This highlights the importance of glycine in collagen, and primary structure to proteins in general.
- Ehlers-Danlos syndrome – deficiency in lysyl oxidase, preventing formation of cross-links between tropocollagen molecules.

1.2.3.2 Histones
In order to condense DNA as much as possible, chromosomes have various levels of packaging, the first levels of which involves the binding of DNA to globular histone proteins, in an approximately 1:1 ratio.

Primary structure – histones are highly basic proteins, with 25% of their amino acids being lysine or arginine. This confers a large positive charge, allowing the protein to bind strongly to the negatively charged phosphate groups of DNA.

Multiprotein complex – there are 5 different types of histone protein involved in chromosome packaging (H1, H2A, H2B, H3 and H4). In chromosomes, octamers form consisting of two molecules each of histones H2A, H2B, H3 and H4. A 146bp long stretch of double-stranded DNA wraps around this octamer, forming a DNA-histone complex known as a nucleosome. Histone H1 sits on the outside of the nucleosome, attached to 'linker' DNA. Interactions between two H1 molecules on adjacent nucleosomes draw the nucleosomes together.

CHAPTER 2

Enzymes and Enzymic Catalysis

2.1 CONCEPTS OF BIOCHEMICAL REACTIONS AND ENZYMES

Catalysis – the acceleration of a chemical reaction by means of a substance that is itself not consumed by the overall reaction. A catalyst provides an alternative route of reaction where the activation energy is lower than the original chemical reaction. Catalysts participate in reactions but are neither reactants nor products of the reaction they catalyze.

Enzyme – an organic catalyst. Enzymes control almost all metabolic reactions, are very specific and highly efficient (able to catalyse many reactions per second). They can be regulated and controlled, and are often proteins but some, such as ribozymes, are not.

2.2 STRUCTURE AND FUNCTION OF ENZYMES

The specificity and activity of enzymes is determined by its active site. This has a particular 3D shape, dependent upon the tertiary protein structure and thus interactions between residues far apart in the polypeptide chain. Hence, the amino acid sequence of an enzyme determines its specificity, as demonstrated by the small residue differences in the active sites of serine protease group enzymes (trypsin, chymotrypsin, elastase) – each cleave peptide bonds in protein substrates, but only some can act on certain proteins.

All active sites have two domains:
- Binding site – holds enzymes and substrate in the correct orientation.
- Catalytic site – area in which reaction takes place.

There are two models for the interaction of enzymes with their substrate:
- Lock and key hypothesis – Emil Fischer, 1894. States that the specificity of an enzyme for a substrate is determined by structural complementation between substrate and enzyme, as in a key fitting into a lock.
- Induced fit hypothesis – Daniel Koshland, 1958. States enzyme function depends on allosteric behaviour, with the binding of a substrate inducing a conformational change in the active site of the enzyme, due to interactions between multiple subunits within the enzyme.

2.2.1 Isoenzymes

Different forms of the same enzyme, which catalyses the same reaction but with different physical and kinetic properties, can exist. These are known as isoenzymes and include lactate dehydrogenase (LDH) and creatine kinase (CK)

Lactate dehydrogenase

Lactate dehydrogenase is an enzyme found in almost all body tissues, but it rarely leaves cells unless there is some form of damage, in which case it may leak into the blood stream. Elevations in LDH level can be measured either in terms of overall level, or by targeting specific isoenzyme forms of it. The overall measurement shows that tissue damage has occurred, but is not specific to the region of the body.

There are 5 different forms of LDH, each of which is relatively specific to certain areas of the body. Thus by testing for the presence of one of these isoenzymes, the exact type of tissue, cell or organ which is damaged can be targeted.

The isoenzymes are:
- LDH-1 which is present in the heart, red cells, renal cortex and germ cells.

18

- LDH-2 which is present in the heart, red blood cells and renal cortex, but to a lesser level than LDH-1. This is also the most abundant form when a complete test is done.
- LDH-3 is present in the lungs and other tissues.
- LDH-4 is present in the white blood cells, lymph nodes, muscle and liver.
- LDH-5 is present in the liver (at higher levels than LDH-4) and in muscle.

LDH tests are used as indicators of the existence and level of severity of acute or chronic tissue damage. They may also be used as a continuous monitor of the progression of a disease or condition, with an ability to target which organs are responsible or failing. LDH used to be used to monitor myocardial infarctions, with a rise, peak and fall in overall LDH levels, and a rise in LDH-1 above the level of LDH-2 as an indicator of the efficiency of treatment (it is also able to differentiate between MI and chest pains caused by other conditions, such as angina). It was occasionally used in conjunction with CK, and more specifically CK-MB, tests. In modern medicine however, this has been replaced by testing for troponin levels which is far more sensitive and specific to heart muscle injury. If tissue or organ damage is suspected, LDH tests are used to determine which areas are involved in conjunction with other tests (e.g. ALT, AST, ALP) and after this it is used to monitor progression of the problem. LDH tests also are used to identify haemolytic anaemia (in which fragile red blood cells rupture, releasing their cytoplasmic contents).

The overall levels and ratio of the different LDH isoenzymes can be used to diagnose certain conditions. Usually the levels will rise, peak and fall within approximately 14 days. Some problems where LDH tests are used include cerebrovascular accident (such as a stroke), pernicious anaemia, kidney diseases, liver disease, pancreatitis and some cancers. Other times at which LDH levels can rise include when large amounts of vitamin C have been ingested, after strenuous exercise, haemolysis of blood and if platelet count increases.

Creatine kinase
Creatine kinase is an enzyme found in the muscle in the heart, brain and in skeletal muscle. CK is essential in the production of ATP within these muscles to allow movement.

It occurs in three major isoenzyme forms:
- CK-MB (which is found mostly in heart muscle)
- CK-BB (which is found mostly in the brain)
- CK-MM (which is found mostly in the heart and other muscles)

In performing the CK test, the levels being measured are those present in muscles (i.e. CK-MB and CK-MM) since the enzyme in the brain hardly ever enters the blood stream. Levels of CK in the blood rise when there is damage to muscle or heart cells. Therefore the test is carried out (particularly for the MB form) when chest pain occurs in patients to see if they have had a heart attack. In the first 4 to 6 hours after the heart attack the CK in the blood begins to rise, reaching its maximum level after 18 to 24 hours. The levels will return to normal after around 2 to 3 days.

The levels of CK actually vary from person to person and race to race. Those who have a larger amount of muscle in their body normally have higher levels of CK, as do African-Americans. The levels of CK also rise temporarily after extended periods of heavy exercise, such as in weightlifting.

2.2.2 Multienzyme complexes

Some enzymes exist as multienzyme complexes (e.g. pyruvate dehydrogenase) allowing more efficient enzyme activity. Existence as multimeric complexes allows regulation of activity:

- Allosteric interactions – see 2.3.1
- Subunit dissociation – e.g. cAMP-dependent protein kinase (protein kinase A) which phosphorylates various metabolic enzymes, altering their function in a hormone-dependent way. PKA is controlled by cAMP - in the absence of cAMP, the kinase is a tetramer of two regulatory and two catalytic subunits, with the regulatory subunits blocking the catalytic centre of the catalytic subunits. Binding of cAMP (cAMP increases within cells in response to certain hormones/signalling) to the regulatory subunits leads to their dissociation from the catalytic subunits, exposing fully active catalytic centres. Downregulation of PKA occurs by a feedback mechanism - one of the substrates that are activated by the kinase is a phosphodiesterase, which converts cAMP to AMP, thus reducing the amount of cAMP that can activate PKA.

2.2.3 Co-factors

Many enzymes need small, non-protein units (called cofactors) to carry out their function properly. These can be either one or more inorganic ions (e.g. Fe^{2+} or Zn^{2+}) or a complex organic molecule known as a coenzyme. When the cofactor is covalently attached to the enzyme, it is known as a prosthetic group.

Some coenzymes do not stay attached to the enzyme all the time, but instead are sequentially bound and released by the enzyme during its catalytic activity. This type of coenzyme includes the NAD^+, $NADP^+$, FAD^+ and FMN, which are particularly important in metabolism. Many coenzymes are derived from vitamin precursors (e.g. NAD^+ and $NADP^+$ are both derived from niacin) and therefore dietary deficiency can upset enzyme activity.

2.2.4 Kinetic parameters

The rate of an enzyme-catalysed reaction (velocity) is fastest at time zero since substrate concentration is maximal, there is no feedback inhibition from the product and equilibrium strongly favours the forward reaction (Le Chatelier's principle). Thus, enzyme velocities, when comparing two reactions, are measured before 10% of the substrate has been used up, giving an approximation for the rate at time zero (called V_0).

V_0 is dependent upon substrate concentration, enzyme concentration as well as temperature and pH (not discussed here):

- Substrate – at low substrate concentrations, a doubling of [S] leads to a doubling in V_0. However, at higher concentrations, the enzyme becomes saturated (i.e. all active sites are used up) and thus increasing [S] has no effect on V_0. Rate of reaction thus becomes dependent on the rate at which product can leave the enzyme active site.
- Enzyme – when the substrate concentration is saturating (i.e. [S] is very high), a doubling of the enzyme concentration leads to a doubling in V_0.

The way in which velocity varies with substrate concentration is described by the Michaelis-Menton equation, which may be plotted as a graph:

$$V_0 = \frac{V_{max} \times [S]}{K_m + [S]}$$

In which:
- V_{max} – maximal velocity
- K_m – the Michaelis constant, which is a measure of the stability of the enzyme-substrate complex. It is calculated from the sum of the rate constants for the breakdown of the enzyme-substrate complex, divided by the constant for its formation. Experimentally it is determined by the substrate concentration at which velocity is half V_{max}. A high K_m demonstrates a weak substrate binding, whilst a low K_m shows a strong substrate binding.

This can be interpreted graphically:

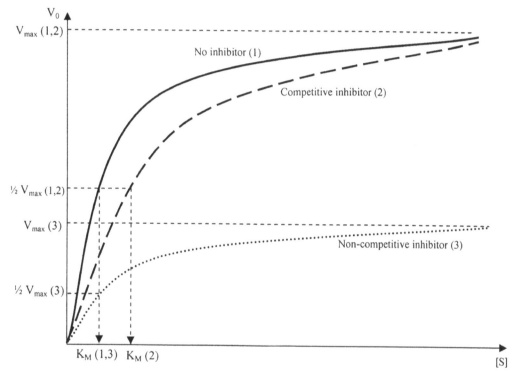

Figure 2.1 – Plot of initial reaction velocity (V_0) against substrate concentration ([S]) under the influence of different inhibitors

As shown above, the effects of various inhibitors can be seen on this plot:
- Competitive – typically structurally similar to the normal substrate for the enzyme and thus competes with the substrate for the active site, to which it binds reversibly. At high [S] the effect of the inhibitor is overcome, and thus **V_{max} does not change, but K_m increases** (an apparent decrease in the affinity of the enzyme for substrate). Examples include competitive inhibition of succinate dehydrogenase by malonate (normal substrate is succinate) and these inhibitors are used widely as drugs due to their temporary effects.
- Non-competitive – inhibitor binds (reversibly) to site other than the active site, leading to a change in the active site. This inhibition is not overcome by an increase in [S] (as no

competition with the inhibitor molecule) and thus V_{max} **falls**. However, K_m **stays the same** since the enzyme still has the same potential affinity for the substrate. An example is the effect of pepstatin on the enzyme renin.

- Irreversible – substances that bind irreversibly, often through a covalent bond, to amino acid residues in or near the active site permanently inactivating the enzyme. Examples include the antibiotic penicillin inhibiting the bacterial cell wall synthase enzyme, or the nerve gas Sarin which inhibits acetylcholinesterase (needed for proper nerve transmission).

2.3 REGULATION OF ENZYME ACTIVITY

Regulation of enzyme activity is essential so that numerous metabolic processes can be coordinated and enzymes made active at the right time, in the right place. Regulation can involve covalent or non-covalent alterations, and occur on various timescales.

2.3.1 Very rapid regulation (seconds)

1. Substrate availability – compartmentalisation
2. Temperature and pH – use in the lab and industry, not within cells
3. Inhibitors – see above
4. Allosteric regulation – often seen in multi-subunit enzymes (with many active sites), where binding of a substrate to one subunit leads to a conformational change, altering the affinity of another site for additional substrate molecules. This is known as co-operative behaviour and, as in haemoglobin, results in a sigmoidal Michaelis-Menton plot. The steep middle section of this curve demonstrates these enzymes are particularly sensitive to small changes in [S] within a narrow physiological range of substrate concentrations. Activity of these enzymes may be regulated by allosteric activators or inhibitors. Examples include aspartate transcarbamoylase, used in pyrimidine synthesis.

2.3.2 Rapid regulation (minutes)

1. Reversible covalent modification – addition or removal of non-protein groups from an enzyme molecule, resulting in changes in tertiary structure and thus catalytic activity. The most common is phosphorylation/dephosphorylation, involving the addition/removal of a phosphate group by kinase/phosphatase enzymes respectively. Various kinases and phosphatases exist, which alter the phosphate groups on specific amino acid residues e.g. serine and threonine protein kinases. Phosphorylation can either increase or decrease the velocity of an enzyme, depending on the enzyme, which is important for the reciprocal regulation of synthesis and breakdown in metabolism. Other modifications include adenylylation, ADP-ribosylation and ubiquitination.
2. Proteolysis – activation of enzymes by cleavage of inactive precursor forms. Particularly important in digestion e.g. pancreatic proteases.

2.3.3 Slow regulation (hours, days, years)

1. Enzyme synthesis – regulation of gene expression by transcription factors, rate of mRNA degradation etc.
2. Enzyme degradation – half-lives of different enzymes vary.

CHAPTER 3

Lipids and Carbohydrates

3.1 LIPIDS

3.1.1 Types of Lipid in the Body
3.1.1.1 Fatty Acids and Glycerides
Fatty acids consist of a hydrocarbon chain with a terminal carboxylic acid group. Most biological fatty acids have an even number of carbon atoms in an unbranched chain (ranging from 14 to 24 carbons normally). The properties of fatty acids, such as their melting points, depend on the chain length (longer = higher melting point) and number of double bonds. Three types of fatty acid exist:
- Saturated – all carbons on the fatty acid chain are saturated with hydrogen atoms.
- Monounsaturated – have one C=C double bond in the chain structure.
- Polyunsaturated – have more than one C=C double bond in the chain, with adjacent double bonds separated by at least one methylene group.

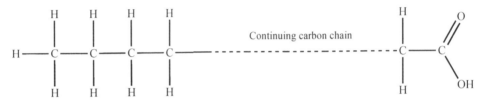
Figure 3.1 – Fatty acid structure

Fats are structures which consist of fatty acids bonded to a backbone structure. This is often glycerol forming a triester known as triacylglycerol. However, other molecules can serve as backbones leading to a wide range of fatty acid containing structures. All fats possess ester bonds between the fatty acid tail and backbone molecule.

Fats are obtained through the diet (particularly from animal products such as meat, milk, eggs) and by synthesis from two-carbon units in the form of acetyl CoA from pyruvate. Essential fatty acids are those that cannot be formed within an organism from other products, and therefore must come from the diet.

3.1.1.2 Phospholipids
Glycerophospholipids are essential molecules for the formation and maintenance of membranes. They are made up of a phosphorylated head group (attached to C-3 of the backbone), a three-carbon glycerol backbone and two fatty acid chains. Although the phosphate group can exist on its own without additional groups bound to it (this is the simplest phospholipid, phosphatidate), most membrane lipids have additional functional groups esterified to the phosphate, such as choline, ethanolamine and another glycerol, which significantly alter their properties.

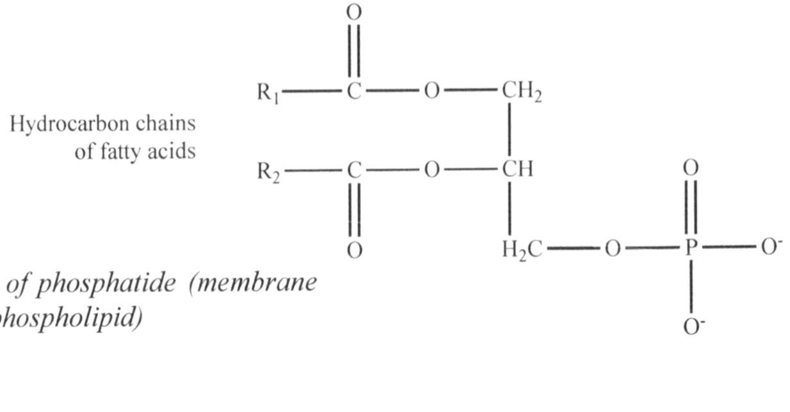

Figure 3.2 – Structure of phosphatide (membrane glycerophospholipid)

3.1.1.3 Sterols
Cholesterol is one of many sterols, and forms an important part of animal plasma membranes, where it regulates fluidity. It contains a system of four fused carbon rings with a short hydrocarbon chain attached to one of the terminal rings. The ring structure imparts rigidity to the molecule.

Cholesterol is an essential precursor for various compounds in the body, including steroid hormones (testosterone, oestrogen, progesterone), bile salts and vitamin D.

3.1.2 Roles of Lipids
Lipids serve a number of roles in the body, for which they are structurally adapted:
- Energy – β-oxidation of fatty acids.
- Structural – act as barriers to diffusion in plasma membranes, as well as stabilising water-fat interfaces (if the lipid is amphipathic) such as with bile salts in the gut, which is essential to fat absorption from the diet, and the formation of lipoproteins for transporting absorbed fats around the body.
- Signalling molecules – extracellular molecules able to influence the function of target cells through receptors, or diffuse into cells and bind to intracellular response elements. Many hormones are steroids e.g. testosterone, aldosterone.

3.2 CARBOHYDRATES

3.2.1 Types of Carbohydrate
Carbohydrates are molecules consisting of carbon, hydrogen and oxygen only.

Monosaccharides (e.g. glucose, fructose, galactose)
Simplest form of carbohydrate, with the general formula $(CH_2O)_n$ where n is 3 or more. Monosaccharides consist of a carbon chain with a number of OH groups attached and either an aldehyde (aldose monosaccharides) or ketone group (ketose monosaccharide). Given the presence of asymmetric carbons, stereoisomers of monosaccharides exist (D and L forms) leading to a range of disaccharides and polysaccharides with different properties.

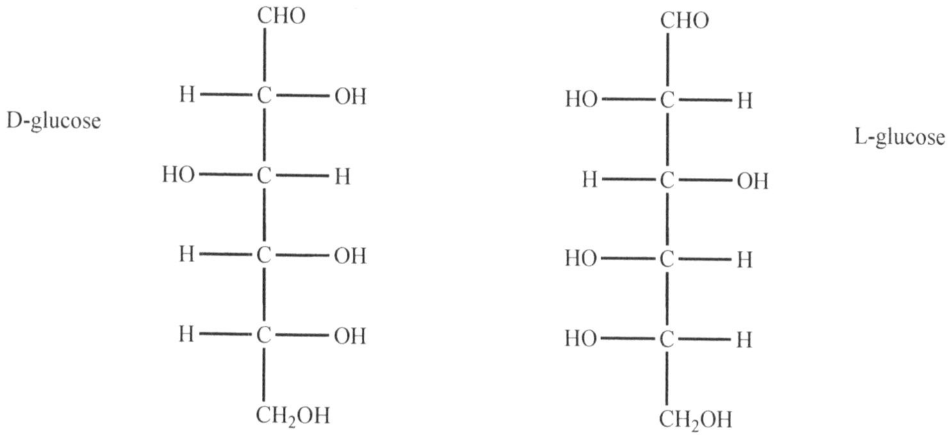

Figure 3.3 – Glucose stereoisomers

The ability of the aldehyde or ketone group to react with an OH group, forming a covalent bond, means monosaccharides can exist in cyclic forms. Six membered ring structures of hexoses (e.g. glucose) are known as pyranoses.

Disaccharides (e.g. sucrose, lactose)
The aldehyde or ketone group on C-1 of a cyclic monosaccharide can react with the OH group on another monosaccharide, forming a disaccharide, joined by a glycosidic link. Glycosidic links are named according to the position of the OH group around the C-1 carbon (α form of a monosaccharide has OH below H on C-1, β other way round) and the carbons on each monosaccharide involved in the bond.

Examples of disaccharides include sucrose (glucose and fructose joined by an α-1,2 link), lactose (glucose and galactose joined by β-1,4 link) and maltose (two glucose joined by an α-1,4 link).

Polysaccharides
Long chains of monosaccharides joined together are known as polysaccharides. Polysaccharide chains may be either linear or branched. They serve many roles in biology, such as energy storage as glycogen in animals (branched glucose polymer, with α-1,4 and α-1,6 links) and as starch in plants (mixture of linear amylase and branched amylopectin – same as glycogen, but with less frequent branching). Cellulose is an unbranching polysaccharide of glucose found in plants, linked by β-1,4 glycosidic bonds.

3.2.2 Roles of Carbohydrates in the Body
3.2.2.1 Structural
Proteoglycans are a major component of the animal extracellular matrix, which exists between cells in an organism. They form large complexes with other proteoglycans, hyaluronan and fibrous matrix proteins (such as collagen). They are also involved in binding cations (such as sodium, potassium and calcium) and water, and regulating the movement of molecules through the matrix.

Proteoglycans represent a special class of glycoproteins that are heavily glycosylated. They consist of a core protein with one or more covalently attached glycosaminoglycan chains. These glycosaminoglycan (GAG) chains are long, linear carbohydrate polymers that are negatively charged under physiological conditions, due to the occurrence of sulphate and acidic groups.

3.2.2.2 Energy Sources
Both animal and plant food sources contain carbohydrates that can be used for energy. Glycogen from animals and starch and cellulose from plants are polysaccharides which can be broken into constituent monosaccharides for glycolysis and eventual ATP production.

Mammals are unable to digest cellulose since they lack enzymes capable of hydrolysing β-1,4 glycosidic links. Ruminants, however, possess large populations of cellulase-producing bacteria in their gut allowing full digestion of grass and other plants.

3.2.2.3 As Biosynthetic Precursors
Carbohydrates are useful in the synthesis of other essential molecules, such as amino acids, fatty acids and nucleotides for nucleic acid synthesis (see later chapters)

3.2.2.4 In Conjugates
Carbohydrates play an essential role in membrane function, forming a protective coat, present as either glycoproteins or glycolipids. They also play a role in intercellular recognition and maintaining

the asymmetry of the membrane (needed for compartmentalisation, diffusion gradients, signalling etc.)

Glycolipids – sugar residues of carbohydrate attached to certain lipids in the membrane (e.g. glycosphingolipids). Some are localised to specific cell types, such as cerebrosides, found mainly in the membrane of neurones. Defects in their formation and metabolism can cause Gaucher's and Krabbe disease.

Glycoproteins – sugar residue of carbohydrate is attached to the polypeptide chains of peripheral or integral membrane proteins. This depends on bonds with the OH group on serine or threonine residues, or the amide (N-C=O) group of asparagine.

CHAPTER 4

Membranes

4.1 SOLUTES, MEMBRANES AND MEMBRANE TRANSPORT

Membranes form boundaries around cells and distinct intracellular compartments, acting as selectively permeable barriers and signal relays. The behaviour of molecules in relation to membranes depends on their size, polarity and charge.

Solubility – refers to the ability for a given substance, the solute, to dissolve in a solvent, measured in terms of the maximum amount of solute dissolved in a solvent at equilibrium. The solvent is often a liquid, water and lipid being the most biologically relevant. The solute can be a gas, another liquid, or a solid.

Osmosis – the net movement of water across a partially permeable membrane from a region of high solvent potential (i.e. less solute, more water) to an area of low solvent potential (i.e. more solute, less water), down a solute concentration gradient. Osmosis is important in biological systems as many biological membranes are partially permeable.

Diffusion – net movement of particles from areas of their higher concentration to areas of their lower concentration until equilibrium is reached.

4.1.1 Transmembrane passage of gases and water

Gases, water and some other molecules (urea, ethanol) are able to pass across lipid bilayers by simple diffusion, a form of passive transport, due to their small uncharged or hydrophobic nature. Since no membrane proteins are involved there is no specificity, with the molecule in aqueous solution on one side of the membrane merely dissolving into the lipid bilayer, crossing it, and dissolving into the aqueous solution on the other side. Thus, rate of movement across the membrane for these molecules is directly proportional to the concentration gradient across the membrane.

4.1.2 Transmembrane passage of ions and substrates

Large uncharged polar molecules (e.g. glucose), ions and charged polar molecules (e.g. ATP, amino acids) are unable to cross membranes passively. They thus require integral membrane proteins to traverse the membrane, and in some cases, the input of energy as well. Membranes are full of a range of channels and carriers to allow transport of these molecules across otherwise impermeable barriers.

4.1.2.1 Channels

Passive transport down a concentration gradient can occur through transmembrane channels, without requiring energy input.

Voltage-gated – class of transmembrane ion channels that are activated by changes in electrical potential difference near the channel. Changes in the potential difference across the channel induces conformational changes, exposing a central pore down which ions (or other molecules) can pass. The channels tend to be ion-specific, although similarly sized and charged ions may also travel through them to some extent. Examples include those for sodium and potassium ions, especially critical in neurons and maintaining the resting membrane potential of all cells.

Ligand-gated – channels that are opened or closed in response to binding of a chemical messenger (ligand) which induces a conformational change in parts of the protein blocking the central pore. The prototypic ligand-gated ion channel is the nicotinic acetylcholine receptor consisting of a pentamer of protein subunits, with two binding sites for ACh. When the ligands bind, they alter the receptor's configuration and cause an internal Na^+-specific pore to open, allowing Na^+ ions to flow down their electrochemical gradient into the cell. With a sufficient number of channels opening at once, the intracellular Na^+ concentration rises to the point at which the positive charge within the cell depolarises the membrane, and an action potential is initiated.

4.1.2.2 Carriers
Carriers do not rely on a central pore, but instead move substances across the membrane by binding them on one side, carrying them across the membrane, and releasing them on the other side. They may be either passive or active.

Primary active transporters – active carriers, which require an input of energy from the coupled hydrolysis of ATP. Hydrolysis of ATP to ADP and P_i by an integral ATPase causes a conformational change allowing the transport of bound ions across the membrane. Arguably the most important is the Na^+/K^+-ATPase, transporting 3 Na^+ out and 2 K^+ into the cell, maintaining concentration gradients and potential difference across the membrane essential for cellular function.

Secondary active transporters – active carriers in which the energy for movement of a molecule comes from ions passing down their concentration gradient, releasing their potential energy. If both the ion and transported molecule pass in the same direction the transporter is a symport, whereas reciprocal movement transporters are antiports. Examples include the Na^+/Ca^{2+} exchange (NCX) antiport which transports one calcium ion out of the cell, for every three sodium ions allowed to pass into the cell. Absorption of glucose in the intestine relies on Na^+/glucose symporter protein, whereby energy released from the passage of sodium down its concentration gradient allows glucose to be taken up into the (relatively high glucose concentration) cytosol of intestinal epithelial cells

Facilitated diffusion – facilitated diffusion does not rely on an input in energy, since ions and molecules pass down their concentration gradients. Binding of transported substances to one side of the membrane (often with another ion or molecule binding on the other side) induces a conformational change in the integral membrane protein, causing transport to the other side of the membrane where it is released. Examples include the Band 3 Cl^-/HCO_3^- exchange protein, present in erythrocytes and the collecting duct of the kidney, important physiologically in the blood-borne transport of CO_2 and pH regulation by the renal system.

4.1.3 Kinetics
Given their ability to bind to specific molecules and ions, carriers display the same Michaelis-Menton kinetics as enzymes. Thus, they possess a V_{max} and K_m, saturating at a certain concentration. Furthermore, they are affected by temperature, pH and inhibitor molecules.

Simple diffusion and passage through channels does not require binding to 'active sites'. Therefore, kinetics for substances moving by this mechanism show linearity, with an increase in concentration leading to a directly proportional increase in rate of movement. Saturation is not possible, as long as a concentration gradient (and cellular integrity) is maintained.

4.2 COMPOSITION OF MEMBRANES
Membranes are made up of lipids, proteins and carbohydrates in various proportions. Each of these groups of molecules serves a specific set of structural and functional roles, and therefore alterations in the relative contribution of each to a membrane has implications for its behaviour.

4.2.1 Lipids
Lipids act as the main structural components of membranes, and fall into three groups. They can also serve as signalling molecules in the membrane.

Glycerophospholipids – membrane lipids consisting of a phosphorylated headgroup, glycerol backbone and two hydrocarbon fatty acid chains. There are various types of glycerophospholipid, which vary in their phosphorylated headgroup.

Sphingolipids – sphingolipids are similar to glycerophospholipids except they have a sphingosine backbone in the place of glycerol. This means that, in addition to the phosphorylated headgroup (as found in glycerophospholipids) they have one fatty acid chain derived from the sphingosine back-bone, and one additional fatty acid chain, attached to the backbone by an amide bond.

Both glycerophospholipids and sphingolipids play a particularly important role in providing the structural foundation to membranes. Since both contain one hydrophobic region and one hydrophilic region (i.e. they are amphipathic) they orientate automatically into lipid bilayers in the presence of water. This relies also on the bulky fatty acid groups of phospholipids, which prevent spherical micelle formation. In addition, certain specific glycerophospholipids and sphingolipids are located in certain cell membranes on account of special features – e.g. sphingomyelins in the insulating myelin sheath around nerve cells, cerebrosides in brain neural cells, cardiolipin (diphosphatidylglycerol) in inner mitochondrial membranes.

Cholesterol – cholesterol is a major component of animal plasma membranes and is more rigid than other membrane lipids, on account of its fused ring structure. Thus, alterations in cholesterol content are used by cells to regulate their membrane fluidity. An increase in cholesterol (in physiological conditions) will decrease the fluidity of the membrane due to the rigid ring structure preventing the movement of fatty acid chains. Membrane fluidity also varies with the length, saturation and *cis/trans* configuration of fatty acid chains in the other lipids.

4.2.2 Proteins
Proteins in the membrane serve a number of functions ranging from transport and signalling to structural integrity and enzymic catalysis in the surrounding medium. Membrane proteins are classi-fied as either intrinsic or extrinsic depending on their mode of attachment to the lipid bilayer. In general, extrinsic proteins are more important for maintaining and altering cell shape, whilst intrinsic proteins are involved in signalling, transport and catalysis.

4.2.3 Carbohydrates
Carbohydrates form an essential part of membranes forming a protective coat, present as either glycoproteins or glycolipids. They also play a role in intercellular recognition and maintaining the asymmetry of the membrane (needed for compartmentalisation, diffusion gradients, signalling etc.)

Glycolipids – sugar residues of carbohydrate attached to certain lipids in the membrane (e.g. gly-cosphingolipids). Some are localised to specific cell types, such as cerebrosides, found mainly in the membrane of neurones. Defects in their formation and metabolism can cause Gaucher's and Krabbe disease.

Glycoproteins – sugar residue of carbohydrate is attached to the polypeptide chains of peripheral or integral membrane proteins. This depends on bonds with the OH group on serine or threonine residues, or the amide (N-C=O) group of asparagine.

4.3 THE FLUID MOSAIC MODEL OF MEMBRANE STRUCTURE
According to Singer and Nicholson (1972), membranes can be considered as mobile two-dimensional structure. The fluidity of membranes described in this Fluid Mosaic Model means lipids and proteins are able to move freely within the plane of either the inner or outer leaflet (rotating or moving

laterally), but they are unable to flip from one leaflet to another. This has implications for membrane function, with receptors embedded in the membrane able to distribute selectively to certain areas, and membrane constituents able to be recycled.

As described above, the fluidity of membrane is dependent mainly upon lipids and cholesterol, and interference from immobile anchored components (e.g. those bound to the cytoskeleton).

4.3.1 Association of proteins with the lipid phase

Membrane proteins are classified as either extrinsic (peripheral) or intrinsic (integral). Extrinsic proteins are only loosely bound to the membrane by non-covalent ionic and hydrogen bonds. Thus, washing membranes with high pH/ionic strength solutions allows these proteins to be removed. Intrinsic proteins however are tightly bound to the membrane through interactions with the hydrophobic core of the bilayer, and can therefore only be extracted with organic solvents or detergents that upset the actual membrane itself.

4.3.1.1 Extrinsic (surface) proteins

Extrinsic proteins can be found on either the inner or outer surface of membranes, associated with the membrane by non-covalent interactions with either the lipid headgroups or other proteins. These proteins are generally water soluble (globular).

Cytoskeleton – extrinsic membrane proteins are used extensively to form the internal cytoskeleton of cells. A network of proteins such as spectrin, actin, Band 4.1 and ankyrin give cells strength and flexibility, thus maintaining cell shape, which is essential for function.

4.3.1.2 Intrinsic proteins

Most intrinsic proteins have one or more regions of polypeptide which span the membrane, interacting with the hydrophobic internal fatty acid chains of the membrane bilayer. Some are also anchored by covalently attached fatty acid or hydrocarbon chains.

Transmembrane proteins – the first evidence of membrane spanning regions anchoring proteins came from the study of glycophorin A in red blood cells. Sequencing the amino acids of this protein revealed the hydrophobic central region that spans the membrane consists mainly of amino acid residues with hydrophobic side chains, arranged into an α-helix. Exposure of hydrophobic amino acids allows them to interact via hydrophobic bonds with the fatty acid chains. Many transmembrane proteins have multiple membrane-spanning α-helices, such that the polypeptide loops backwards and forwards through the membrane (helices joined by short, surface-exposed hydrophilic regions). Examples of this include G-proteins, important in signal transduction that cross the membrane 7 times, and anion exchange band 3 protein in erythrocytes, crossing the membrane 12-14 times.

Lipid-anchored proteins – some intrinsic proteins are anchored in the cell membrane by covalent association with a hydrocarbon chain, which, being hydrophobic, is able to embed itself in the membrane. Multiple lipid anchors are used, such as GPI, myristate and palmitate. Examples of lipid-anchored proteins include the enzyme alkaline phosphatase.

4.4 FUNCTIONS OF MEMBRANE PROTEINS

4.4.1 Transport through Lipid Membranes

See 4.1.3.2.

4.4.2 Vesicular Transport

Vesicles are relatively small and enclosed compartments, separated from the cytosol by at least one lipid bilayer. The membrane enclosing the vesicle is similar to that of the plasma membrane allowing the internal environment to be different from that in the cytosol. Vesicles store, transport, or digest cellular products and waste and are a basic tool of the cell for organizing metabolism, transport, enzyme storage, as well as being chemical reaction chambers. Many vesicles are made in the Golgi apparatus, but also in the endoplasmic reticulum, or from parts of the plasma membrane. Vesicles are able to move between compartments in the cell, as is seen with the release of neurotransmitter from vesicles which travel from neuron-internal areas to the synapse.

Formation and targeting of vesicles

Vesicle formation is dependent on membrane proteins, and their interactions with other surface proteins and the substances to be transported. The assembly of a vesicle requires numerous coats to surround and bind to the substances being transported. A family of coats are called adaptins, bind to the coat vesicle trapping various transmembrane receptor proteins, called cargo receptors, which in turn trap the cargo molecules. As such, the combinations of different receptor proteins on the surface of the vesicle determine its contents.

Movement of vesicles is controlled by motor proteins. Alterations in protein conformation lead to motion along a defined 'track'. Often, this involves cytoskeletal elements such as microtubules (as used to move and split chromosomes in mitosis and meiosis). Subsequent, protein surface markers on vesicles (v-SNAREs) interact with complementary t-SNAREs on the target membranes to cause fusion of the vesicle and target membrane. Rab protein (regulatory GTP-binding protein) is thought to control the binding of these complementary SNAREs ensuring the correct vesicles traffic to the correct place.

There are three types of vesicle coats: clathrin, COPI and COPII, each with their own targeting pathways.
- Clathrin coats are found on vesicles trafficking between the Golgi and plasma membrane, the Golgi and endosomes, and the plasma membrane and endosomes.
- COPI coated vesicles are responsible for retrograde transport from the Golgi to the ER
- COPII coated vesicles are responsible for anterograde transport from the ER to the Golgi.

Fusion requires the two membranes to be brought within 1.5 nm of each other. For this to occur water must be displaced from the surface of the vesicle membrane. This is energetically unfavourable, and evidence suggests that the process requires ATP, GTP and acetyl-CoA.

CHAPTER 5

Subcellular Organelles, the Nucleus and Trafficking

5.1 SUB-CELLULAR ORGANELLES

Eukaryotic cells are bounded by a plasma membrane and contain a membrane-bounded nucleus, along with other organelles. Organelles are always membrane bound, allowing enclosure of a specific complement of proteins and other molecules such that they can perform a particular role. As described in chapter 4 the plasma membrane is essential for maintaining ionic composition and osmolarity of the cytosol by being selectively permeable, and also plays roles in communication with other cells, endocytosis and exocytosis, catalysis in the external environment etc.

5.1.1 Rough endoplasmic reticulum

Structure – interconnected network of membrane vesicles studded with ribosomes on the cytosolic surface.

Function – the ribosomes on RER are the sites of membrane and secretory protein biosynthesis. Within the lumen of the RER are enzymes which are involved in post-translational modifications (e.g. glycosylation, cleavage of long precursors) of newly synthesised proteins, essential to their function.

5.1.2 Smooth endoplasmic reticulum

Structure – interconnected network of membrane vesicles without ribosome studding.

Function – SER is involved in phospholipid biosynthesis, and also certain detoxification reactions.

5.1.3 Ribosomes

Structure – 20nm in diameter and are composed of 65% ribosomal RNA and 35% ribosomal proteins. Consist of small and large subunits, each of which is a multicomponent complex of rRNA and protein. Large subunits (60S) contain three rRNAs (28S, 5.8S and 5S) complexed with 49 polypeptides. Small subunits (40S) consist of 18S rRNA and 33 polypeptides. They may be cytosol-free or membrane bound.

Function – central to protein biosynthesis, translating messenger RNA (mRNA) into protein. mRNA comprises a series of codons that dictate the sequence of the amino acids needed to make the protein. Using the mRNA as a template, the ribosome traverses each codon of the mRNA, pairing it with the appropriate amino acid using transfer RNA (tRNA) containing a complementary anti-codon on one end and the appropriate amino acid on the other.

5.1.4 Golgi apparatus

Structure – system of flattened membrane-bound sacs, able to fuse with vesicles from the RER.

Function – obtain membrane and secretory proteins from the RER via vesicle migration and fusion, and subsequently performs further post-translational modifications on the proteins. Also, signal sequences and tags are used to 'sort' the proteins in vesicles, which then move through the cytosol to appropriate organelles.

5.1.5 Mitochondria

Structure – double membrane-bound organelle, with a space between the two membranes. The outer membrane is permeable to many molecules on account of porin channels. The inner membrane is much less permeable, with large infoldings (cristae) protruding into the central matrix. The central matrix contains mitochondrial DNA, along with various enzymes and proteins.

Function – inner membrane is the site of oxidative phosphorylation and electron transport, synthesising ATP. The central matrix is the site of numerous metabolic reactions e.g. Kreb's cycle.

5.1.6 Lysosomes
Structure – single membrane-bound organelles, with proton pumps in their membrane for maintaining a low internal pH.

Function – have a mildly acidic pH (around pH 4-5) and a range of hydrolases which are fully active in acid conditions (acid hydrolases). The combination of enzymes and acid is used to degrade host and foreign macromolecules (e.g. proteases break down polypeptides, lipases lipids, nucleases DNA and RNA) and substances internalised by endocytosis.

5.1.7 Cytoskeleton
The cytosol (cytoplasm without organelles) of eukaryotic cells contains an internal scaffold known as the cytoskeleton, which maintains the shape of the cell and moves vesicles/organelles around. The cytoskeleton is composed of three different types of filament.

Microtubules
Structure – hollow cylindrical structures with a diameter of 30nm, composed of tubulin protein. The wall of the microtubule cylinder is composed of a helical array of α- and β-tubulin subunits.

Function – form supportive framework along which subcellular organelles move within the cytosol. This is particularly important in processes such as cell division, where paired replicated chromosomes are separated to opposite poles of the cell. Microtubule poisons (e.g. taxol – Docetaxel, Paclitaxel) are used to prevent the rapid, uncontrolled cell division seen in cancer.

Intermediate filaments
Structure – 7-11nm in diameter, and can be composed of various different proteins depending on the cell (e.g. keratin, desmin, nestin are all intermediate filament proteins).

Function – generally involved in load-bearing function within cells, such as the keratin intermediate filament network, found in the skin of animals.

Microfilaments
Structure – approximately 7nm in diameter, and composed of actin.

Function – play a role in mechanical support. They can interact with myosin to form contractile elements, which can move various bits of the cell e.g. form membrane invaginations for endocytosis.

5.2 THE NUCLEUS

5.2.1 Size and Structure
The nucleus is the largest cellular organelle, with an average diameter typically varying from 11 to 22μm and occupying about 10% of the total volume in mammalian cells.

The main structural elements of the nucleus are the nuclear envelope, a double membrane that encloses the entire organelle and keeps its contents separated from the cellular cytoplasm, the nuclear lamina, a meshwork within the nucleus that adds mechanical support, much like the cytoskeleton supports the cell as a whole and the nucleolus. The outer nuclear membrane is often continuous with RER to allow efficient protein transcription and translation.

The nuclear membrane is impermeable to most molecules and thus nuclear pores are required to allow movement of molecules across the envelope. These pores represent points where the two membranes fuse, providing a channel that allows free movement of small molecules and ions. The movement of larger molecules, such as proteins, is carefully controlled, and requires active transport facilitated by carrier proteins. Nuclear transport is of paramount importance to cell function, as movement through the pores is required for both gene expression and chromosomal maintenance.

Although the interior of the nucleus does not contain any membrane-delineated bodies, its contents are not uniform. A number of sub-nuclear bodies exist, made up of unique proteins, RNA molecules, and DNA conglomerates. The most important of these is the nucleolus, which is mainly involved in assembly of ribosomes.

5.2.2 Nuclear Functions
The nucleus contains most of a cell's genetic material – DNA packaged with histone proteins forming chromosomes. As such, the nucleus is essential in gene replication, repair and transcription.

In addition, the nucleolus represents the subnuclear body where ribosomes are synthesised. The nucleolus is roughly spherical, and is surrounded by a layer of condensed chromatin, although no membrane separates it from the other nuclear contents. Nucleoli are made of protein and ribosomal DNA (rDNA) sequences present on chromosomes 13, 14, 15, 21 and 22. Transcription of rDNA in the nucleolus initiates the formation of ribosomes, providing not only the rRNA, but also polypeptides present in the small and large subunits, and signal molecules/transcription factors for their assembly.

5.2.3 The Interphase Nucleus
Interphase is the part of the cell cycle defined only by the absence of cell division during which the cell obtains nutrients, and duplicates its chromatids – each chromosome consists of a pair of chromatids joined by a centromere. During interphase, the chromosome material is in the form of loosely coiled threads called chromatin. There are two types of interphase chromatin – euchromatin and heterochromatin, which vary in density and therefore affect transcription of genes contained within them.

5.2.3.1 Euchromatin
This is a lightly packed form of chromatin that is often (but not always) under active transcription. Euchromatin is reminiscent of an unfolded set of beads along a string, with beads representing nucleosomes around which the wrapping is loose so that the raw DNA may be accessed. It is believed that the presence of methylated lysine on the tails of histone acts as a general marker for euchromatin, allowing unpacking.

Euchromatin participates in the active transcription of DNA with the unfolded structure allowing regulatory proteins and RNA polymerase complexes to bind to the DNA sequence. There is a direct link between how actively productive a cell is and the amount of euchromatin that can be found in its nucleus. It is thought that the cell uses transformation from euchromatin into heterochromatin as a method of controlling gene expression and replication, since such processes behave differently on densely compacted chromatin – this is known as the `accessibility hypothesis'.

5.2.3.2 Heterochromatin
Heterochromatin is a densely packed form of DNA in which transcription is limited. Heterochromatin serves to regulate gene expression and protect the integrity of chromosomes, both of these roles can be attributed to the dense packing of DNA making it less accessible to DNA-binding factors.

Constitutive – all cells of a given species will package the same regions of DNA in constitutive (constantly tightly packed) heterochromatin, and thus in all cells any genes contained within the constitutive heterochromatin will be poorly expressed. For example, all human chromosomes 1, 9, 16, and the Y chromosome contain large regions of constitutive heterochromatin. In most organisms, constitutive heterochromatin occurs around the chromosome centromere and near telomeres.

Facultative – the regions of DNA packaged in facultative (packaging varies over time) heterochromatin will not be consistent across cells within a species. Thus, a sequence in one cell that is packaged in facultative heterochromatin (and the genes within poorly expressed) may be packaged in euchromatin in another cell (with potential to be expressed). The formation of facultative heterochromatin is regulated, and is often associated with morphogenesis or differentiation. An example of facultative heterochromatin is X-chromosome inactivation in female mammals – one X chromosome is packaged in facultative heterochromatin and silenced (forming a Barr body), whilst the other is packaged in euchromatin and expressed.

5.2.4 Nuclear Membrane and Pores

The presence of a double-membrane around the nucleus defines eukaryotes. The membrane is studded with pores, through which molecules can pass in either direction. There are on average 2000 nuclear pore complexes in the nuclear envelope of a vertebrate cell, performing up to 1000 translocations per second each. The entire pore complex has a diameter of about 120 nm, the diameter of the opening is around 50 nm and its depth is about 200 nm. The proteins that make up the nuclear pore complex are known as nucleoporins.

In general, mRNA, proteins and ribosomes pass out of the nucleus, whilst other proteins such as those involved in gene regulation pass in. Although smaller molecules simply diffuse through the pores, larger molecules may be recognized by specific signal sequences (Nuclear Localisation Signals and Nuclear Export Signals) and then enter or exit the nucleus with the help of nucleoporins.

5.3 TRAFFICKING

After synthesis of protein precursors on the ribosomes of the RER, or free in the cytoplasm, vesicle trafficking allows post-translational modifications and targeting to appropriate areas.

ER to Golgi apparatus – allows passage through these two organelles, with initial synthesis of the protein at the ribosomes on the RER and post-translational modifications in its lumen. Subsequent passage to the Golgi (vesicles bud off from RER, pass to Golgi using microtubules, fuse with Golgi) allows additional modifications and 'sorting' according to signal molecules on the protein.

Golgi to plasmalemma/lysosomes – vesicles budding off from the Golgi, containing groups of proteins targeted either to the cell membrane or lysosomes (proteolysis of pre-cursors into active proteins). Integral membrane proteins trafficking to the plasmalemma will add material to it (i.e. vesicle fuses with the cell membrane such that membrane-integral proteins of the vesicle become part of the cell membrane). Those proteins contained within the vesicle lumen are secreted into the extracellular space when the vesicle membrane fuses with the cell membrane. This can be continuous and non-regulated, or regulated according to prevailing conditions e.g. neurotransmitter release at synapses on depolarisation of neurone membrane, release of insulin from β-cells in response to glucose levels. Substances which are secreted in a regulated fashion are stored in the cytoplasm in clathrin-coated vesicles which bud off from the Golgi.

5.3.1 Receptor-mediated endocytosis

Receptor-mediated endocytosis is the process by which cells internalize molecules by the inward budding of plasma membrane in response to cell membrane receptors specific to the molecule. This occurs at clathrin-coated pits at the membrane, forming clathrin-coated vesicles. Receptor-mediated endocytosis allows the selective concentration of particular macromolecules which are at a low concentration in the extracellular fluid. This increases the efficiency of uptake without being dependent on high extracellular concentrations.

Binding of extracellular macromolecules to their membrane-bound receptors leads to accumulation of receptor-macromolecule complexes at clathrin-coated pits in the membrane. The recruitment of receptor-macromolecule complexes in turn increases the polymerisation of clathrin protein at the intracellular face of the membrane, which causes the membrane to bud inwards. Once sufficient clathrin has been polymerised, the membrane buds inwards completely, forming a vesicle coated in a clathrin cage, containing receptor-macromolecule complexes. Subsequently, the vesicle moves through the cytosol and sheds its coat (becoming early endosomes) maturing into late endosomes, which pass to lysosomes. Enzymes in the lysosome separate the receptor from its macromolecule. Receptors will be recycled to the membrane, whilst the macromolecule will either be released into the cytosol or trafficked to another organelle.

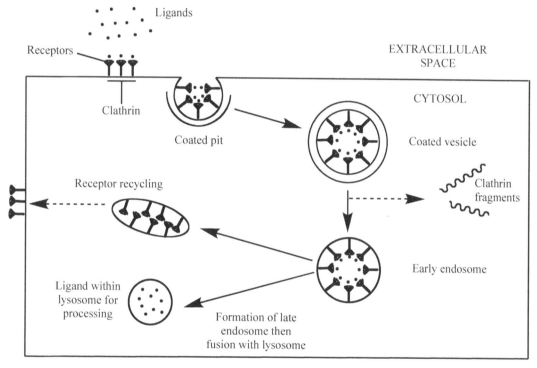

Figure 5.1 – Receptor-mediated endocytosis

This process of uptake is used by mammalian cells to take up cholesterol. However, disease causing organisms such as viruses (e.g. smallpox virus Vaccinia) and toxins produced by other organisms can also gain access to target cells in this way, 'hijacking' this physiologically important pathway.

5.3.2 Transcytosis
Transcytosis is the transport of macromolecular cargo from one side of a cell to the other within a membrane-bounded carrier i.e. vesicle. It is a strategy used by multicellular organisms to selectively move material between two different environments while maintaining the distinct compositions of

those environments. Vesicles are employed to intake the macromolecules on one side of the cell, draw them through it, and eject them on the other side.

This process is most commonly observed in cells forming an epithelium, such as in the gut, where uptake of food macromolecules can occur through transcytosis, whilst antibodies (IgA) are exported into the gut lumen to protect against microorganisms. Blood capillaries are another well recognised and important site for transcytosis.

Transcytotic cargo is not thought to be limited to macromolecules, with several vitamins and ions utilising endocytic mechanisms and vesicular carriers as part of their transcellular pathway.

CHAPTER 6

Cellular Metabolism – General Principles

6.1 GENERAL PRINCIPLES

The overall strategy of human metabolism is to gain energy from food substances, with macromolecules being partially or completely oxidised, resulting in the reduction of co-factors or direct production of ATP/GTP. This involves various enzymes and is tightly regulated, taking place in specialised areas within the cell (i.e. mitochondria and other organelles). Subsequently, the potential energy stored in the reduced co-factors is released, with the phosphorylation of ADP to ATP. ATP is known as the 'energy currency' of the cell, and as such any energy-requiring reaction is linked to its hydrolysis back to ADP. Metabolism of any macromolecule involves the release of water and CO_2.

6.1.1 Principles of Metabolic Control

In order that metabolism occurs in the right place, at the right time and is maximally efficient, enzymes and transporter molecules integral to it are tightly regulated. As with enzyme regulation discussed before, this can occur on a short or long-term basis. Note the principles described below are just that – principles – and the details of regulation of specific enzymes are dealt with later.

Enzyme control
Short-term controls:
- Allosteric effects (milliseconds)
- Covalent modification (seconds to minutes)

Long-term controls:
- Enzyme induction/suppression by regulating transcription and translation (hours to days)

Cycles between organs
Although all cells in the body undergo metabolism to some degree, certain organs are specialised for performing particular metabolic roles. This is especially true for the liver. As such, it is necessary to have cycles between organs, allowing substrates to be used in appropriate places. The movement of substances between organs demonstrates that the control of metabolism extends beyond merely

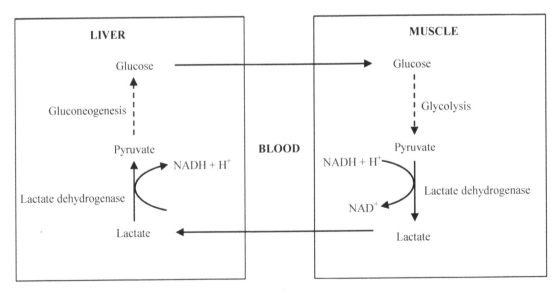

Figure 6.1 – The Cori cycle

regulating enzymes, including the delivery (often dependent on functioning circulation) and trans-membrane movement (dependent on diffusion gradients or membrane transports) of substrates.

The Cori cycle is a perfect example of organ cycling. During vigorous exercise, oxygen levels are low. Thus, the formation of NADH by glycolysis (occurring at normal speed) outstrips the ability of the electron transport chain to oxidise it back to NAD^+ (a process that requires oxygen at the final step – see later). To overcome this, pyruvate, the end product of glycolysis, is converted to lactate by lactate dehydrogenase generating NAD^+. NAD^+ is used early in glycolysis and thus maintaining high levels of it allow complete passage of glucose to pyruvate, generating 2 molecules of ATP in the absence of oxygen.

However, lactate is a dead-end product, and cannot be used by the muscle cells where it was produced, unless it is converted back into pyruvate. Thus, lactate diffuses and is transported out of the muscle cells, into the circulation and passes to the liver. The liver then actively and passively takes up lactate and, given the presence of necessary enzymes, converts it back to pyruvate and subsequently glucose by gluconeogenesis. The glucose is then released from the liver to be used by the skeletal tissue and brain. This process occurs most rapidly in anaerobic conditions, both by nature of the high level of lactate and the specific regulation of transporters (and circulation) necessary for lactate mobilisation.

6.1.2 Oxidation-Reduction Reactions

In reduction-oxidation reactions, the oxidation of a molecule involves the loss of electrons, whilst the reduction of it involves the gain of electrons. Since electrons cannot be destroyed, the oxidation of one molecule must result in the reduction of another. This is the basis for storage of potential energy in metabolism, and the subsequent synthesis of ATP or GTP.

Oxidation and reduction in human metabolism are carried out using $NAD^+/NADH$, $FAD/FADH_2$ and $NADP^+/NADPH$, where NAD^+, FAD and $FADP^+$ are the oxidised forms and thus have the potential to oxidise a substrate.

Oxidation of water, reduction of NAD^+

$$NAD^+ + H_2O \quad \rightarrow \quad NADH + H^+ + \tfrac{1}{2}O_2$$

Oxidation of NADH, reduction of O_2

$$NADH + H^+ + \tfrac{1}{2}O_2 \quad \rightarrow \quad NAD^+ + H_2O$$

The metabolism of molecules in cells results in the storage of energy as potential energy, which must be utilised to synthesise ATP. The TCA cycle, glycolysis and fatty acid oxidation all lead to the generation potential energy in the form of reduced co-factors – NADH (approximately 52.6 kcal/mol), NADPH and $FADH_2$. Re-oxidation of these co-factors through the electron transport chain and oxidative phosphorylation leads to ATP synthesis.

6.1.3 Role and Control of the TCA Cycle

The TCA (citric acid or Krebs) cycle is used to oxidise pyruvate, formed from the breakdown of glucose, into CO_2 and H_2O. In addition, it oxidises acetyl CoA produced from fatty acid degradation and amino acid degradation, and produces precursors for biosynthetic pathways. Thus, the TCA cycles is the final common pathway for the oxidation of fuel molecules, creating CO_2 and reduced coenzymes, which can be used to synthesise ATP through the electron transport chain.

The TCA cycle takes place in the mitochondrial matrix of eukaryotes, and the cytosol of prokaryotes. Succinate dehydrogenase is the only membrane embedded enzyme involved in the cycle, present in the inner mitochondrial membrane (plasma membrane of prokaryotes).

6.1.3.1 The Cycle
The TCA cycle forms the central part to a three-part cycle in which organic molecules are oxidised to CO_2, producing ATP.

Step 1 – Oxidation of fuel molecules to acetyl CoA
Acetyl CoA is the only substrate of the TCA cycle, and thus fuel molecules must eventually be converted to it to enter the cycle. Some molecules may be directly oxidised to acetyl CoA, such as pyruvate (mainly from glycolysis) which is oxidised by pyruvate dehydrogenase using NAD^+ (reduced to NADH). This also produces CO_2, meaning the reaction is called oxidative decarboxylation.

Carbon skeletons of amino acids and odd chain length fatty acids must leave the cycle and re-enter as acetyl CoA via a phosphoenolpyruvate intermediate, which may subsequently be converted to pyruvate.

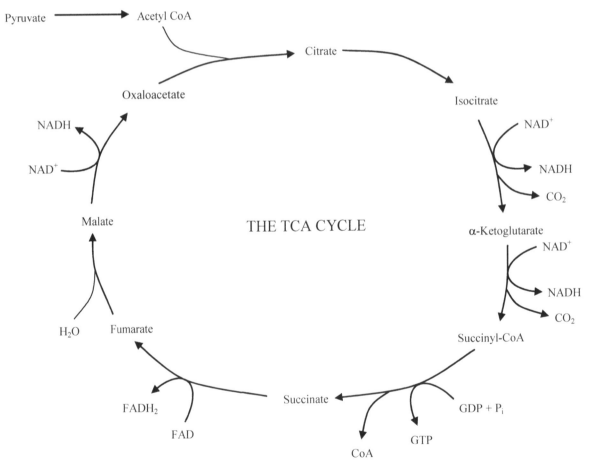

Figure 6.2 – The TCA cycle

Step 2 – The TCA cycle
The TCA cycle oxidises the acetyl groups from acetyl CoA to CO_2, releasing four pairs of electrons, 'stored' as reduced coenzymes NADH and $FADH_2$. There are eight stages.

1. Citrate (6C) is formed from the condensation of acetyl CoA (2C) and oxaloacetate (4C) catalysed by citrate synthase.
2. Citrate is converted to isocitrate (6C) by an isomerisation reaction catalysed by aconitase.
3. Isocitrate is oxidised to α-ketoglutarate (5C) and CO_2 by isocitrate dehydrogenase, using NAD^+ which is reduced to NADH.
4. α-ketoglutarate is oxidised to succinyl CoA (4C) and CO_2 by α-ketoglutarate dehydrogenase, again using NAD^+ as a cofactor, producing the reduced form.
5. Succinyl CoA is converted to succinate (4C) by succinyl CoA synthetase, synthesising one molecule of GTP from GDP and inorganic phosphate in the process, and releasing CoA.
6. Succinate is oxidised to fumarate (4C) by succinate dehydrogenase, reducing FAD to $FADH_2$.
7. Fumarate is converted to malate (4C) by fumarase, requiring the addition of water since this is a hydration reaction.
8. Malate is oxidised to oxaloacetate (4C) by malate dehydrogenase, again producing one molecule of NADH from NAD^+

Step 3 – Oxidation of NADH and $FADH_2$ produced by the TCA cycle
The reduced cofactors produced by the cycle are reoxidised in the electron transport chain, coupled to the phosphorylation of ADP to ATP. Given the use of oxygen as the last electron acceptor in the electron transport chain, the cycle only operates in aerobic conditions, which provide a fresh supply of NAD^+ and FAD.

6.1.3.2 The Products of the Cycle
In addition to the intermediates which may be used elsewhere (see below) the cycle produces:
- 3 NADH (yielding 2.5 ATP each)
- 1 $FADH_2$ (yielding 1.5 ATP)
- 1 GTP

Thus, the oxidation of one acetyl CoA molecule via the TCA cycle produces 12 ATP molecules.

6.1.3.3 Significance of the Cycle
The use of a cycle and not a linear pathway for the oxidation of acetyl CoA serves a catalytic effect. Only small amounts of cycle intermediates are needed to oxidise large amounts of acetyl CoA, since they are constantly being regenerated (i.e. at any one time, the concentration of each intermediate is actually very low). Inhibition of succinate dehydrogenase converts the cycle into a linear pathway, and stoichiometric analysis shows oxidation of one acetyl CoA requires one molecule of oxaloacetate, further demonstrating the existence of the cycle.

6.1.3.4 Connection to Other Pathways
The TCA cycle is connected to other metabolic pathways, both through substrates (e.g. acetyl CoA) and intermediates (e.g. α-ketoglutarate) from the breakdown of macromolecules feeding into it. As such, there is more than one way to use the cycle to synthesis ATP from the products of metabolism (i.e. entering through acetyl CoA).

In addition, intermediates of the cycle can be used to synthesise other substances:
- Citrate – used to synthesise fatty acids.
- α-ketoglutarate – transaminated to allow amino acid and nucleotide synthesis.

- Oxaloacetate – can be converted into glucose via gluconeogenesis, and used to synthesise nucleotides.
- Succinyl CoA – important precursor in the synthesis porphyrin rings in haem groups, essential for haemoglobin, myoglobin and chlorophyll.

If intermediates are drawn off for the synthesis of other molecules, they must be replaced since. Even though they exist at very low catalytic levels, the cycle will cease without the presence of a small amount of each intermediate. Thus, anapleurotic reactions are used:
- Transamination – conversion of glutamate to α-ketoglutarate and aspartate, and subsequently oxaloacetate.
- Pyruvate carboxylase – replenishes oxaloacetate through its formation from pyruvate. Requires biotin cofactor, with pyruvate carboxylase activated by acetyl CoA. High levels of acetyl CoA signal insufficient levels of oxaloacetate to 'use it up' and thus more is synthesised from pyruvate.

6.1.3.5 Regulation of the TCA Cycle
The TCA cycle is regulated according to demand for ATP and not substrate availability. Four enzymes in the cycle are controlled – pyruvate dehydrogenase, citrate synthase, isocitrate dehydrogenase and α-ketoglutarate dehydrogenase. Overall, the cycle increases when energy levels are low, but slows down as ATP accumulates.

Enzyme	Activates	Inhibits
Citrate synthase		Citrate ATP (raises K_M for acetyl CoA)
Isocitrate dehydrogenase	ADP Increased intra-mitochondrial Ca^{2+} concentration	NADH ATP
α-ketoglutarate dehydrogenase	Increased intra-mitochondrial Ca^{2+} concentration	Succinyl CoA NADH
Pyruvate dehydrogenase	Dephosphorylation*	Acetyl CoA NADH Phosphorylation*

* Pyruvate dehydrogenase is also controlled by the balance between phosphorylation and dephosphorylation, performed by kinase and phosphatase enzymes. Increasing NADH, acetyl CoA and ATP stimulates the kinase, thus increasing pyruvate dehydrogenase phosphorylation and inhibiting the enzyme. Conversely, high levels of NAD^+, CoA and ADP increase the activity of the phosphatase. A build up of pyruvate inhibits the kinase, activates the phosphatase and thus stimulates pyruvate conversion to acetyl CoA.

6.1.4 ATP Production and Its Control

ATP is the universal currency of free energy in biological systems, releasing large amounts of energy on hydrolysis to ADP or AMP, which can be harnessed. The phosphoanhydride bond in ATP is neither the least nor most energetic of the phosphate bonds. This intermediate position means reactions in cells release enough energy to synthesise the bond, and yet its hydrolysis also releases sufficient energy to power various processes.

The total quantity of ATP in the human body at any one time is approximately 0.1 mole. The majority of ATP is not usually synthesised de novo, but is generated from ADP. Thus, at any given time, the intracellular concentration of ATP remains constant.

The energy used by human cells requires the hydrolysis of 100 to 150 moles of ATP daily, which equates to 50 to 75 kg, whilst less than 100g is stored at any one time. This means that each ATP molecule is recycled 1000 to 1500 times during a single day.

The cytoplasmic concentration of ATP is ~5mM, whilst that of ADP is ~10μM. Since ATP concentration does not change significantly during metabolic activity, the signal of ATP utilisation is increasing ADP. In addition, since ADP is present at a much lower concentration than ATP, it is a much more sensitive indicator – a change of 1μM represents 10%.

ATP production involves:
1. Generation of reduced co-factors through metabolism of energy substrates.
2. Use of reduced co-factors to generate a proton gradient across mitochondrial membranes.
3. Discharge of the proton gradient, coupled to the formation of ATP.

In addition, ATP and GTP may be synthesised at the level of substrate metabolism (e.g. glycolysis, TCA cycle).

6.1.5 Pathways of Mitochondrial Oxidation

6.1.5.1 The Electron Transport Chain

The oxidation of reduced cofactors releases a large amount of energy that can be used to synthesise ATP. However, these two processes are not directly linked, and instead electrons from reduced co-factors (NADH and $FADH_2$) are passed down a series of electron carriers, finally reaching oxygen, forming water. This is known as the electron transport chain, which is a stepwise sequence of redox reactions with increasing redox potentials, releasing energy at each stage which is used to create a proton gradient (see below).

The electron transport chain consists of three large protein complexes embedded in the inner mito-chondrial membrane (NADH dehydrogenase, cytochrome bc_1 complex and cytochrome oxidase), linked by two small electron carriers (ubiquinone (coenzyme Q) and cytochrome c). The three large protein complexes consist of several electron carriers, which work sequentially to carry electrons down the chain.

NADH to NADH dehydrogenase

NADH dehydrogenase consists of over 30 polypeptides. It binds to NADH and reoxidises it to NAD^+ releasing two electrons:
1. Two electrons from NADH pass to prosthetic group FMN (flavin mononucleotide), creating $FMNH_2$ – each electron is also accepted with a proton.

2. Electrons then transferred within the NADH dehydrogenase complex to FeS (iron-sulphur) clusters in FeS proteins – within FeS clusters an electron is carried by iron ions, which are reduced from Fe^{3+} to Fe^{2+}.
3. Electrons in the $Fe^{2+}S$ clusters are passed to the next electron carrier complex, oxidising back to $Fe^{3+}S$.

NADH dehydrogenase to CoQ
CoQ is a small lipid-soluble molecule in the inner mitochondrial membrane. It acts as an electron carrier, accepting two electrons and two H^+ from NADH dehydrogenase thus being converted to $CoQH_2$.

CoQ to cytochrome bc_1 complex
$CoQH_2$ donates its two electrons and two H^+ to the cytochrome bc_1 complex. This complex of electron carriers contains two cytochromes – cytochrome b and c_1 – plus an FeS containing protein. Cytochromes are defined as proteins bound to an iron-containing haem group, and all are able to act as electron carriers on account of the Fe^{2+}-Fe^{3+} interchange. Within the cytochrome bc_1 complex the electrons and protons are carried first by cytochrome b, then the FeS protein and finally cytochrome c_1.

The stoichiometry of this set of transfers is complicated, since $CoQH_2$ carries two electron and two H^+, whereas cytochromes can only accept one of each at any time. Thus, transfer occurs in two steps, with the formation of $COQH\cdot$ in between.

Cytochrome bc_1 complex to cytochrome c to cytochrome oxidase
Cytochrome c, the second small electron carrier, resides on the outer surface of the inner mitochondrial membrane. Again, this uses Fe^{2+} and Fe^{3+} transitions to accept the electrons from cytochrome bc_1 and subsequently donate it to cytochrome oxidase.

Cytochrome oxidase to oxygen
Cytochrome oxidase contains two cytochromes (a and a_3) which, in addition to containing iron ions, possess copper atoms which cycle between Cu^{2+} and Cu^+. This additional complexity allows the transfer of four electrons and four H^+ ions to molecular oxygen, with the formation of two molecules of water, completing the electron transport chain.

Electron transport from FADH2
In addition to NADH, some reactions of the TCA cycle produce the reduced co-factor $FADH_2$. In particular, the oxidation of succinate to fumarate in the TCA cycle, by succinate dehydrogenase, results in the production of $FADH_2$. As with NADH, this can be re-oxidised, releasing energy for proton transport.

$FADH_2$ is re-oxidised by succinate-CoQ reductase (complex II) which is an integral inner mitochondrial membrane complex, containing both succinate dehydrogenase and FeS clusters. During re-oxidation of $FADH_2$, two electrons are passed from the reduced cofactor to FeS clusters, and subsequently to ubiquinone (CoQ) allowing them to enter the main electron transport chain. As with NADH, this results in the export of protons. In addition to picking up $FADH_2$ from the TCA cycle, complex II also receives $FADH_2$ from fatty acid oxidation and the glycerol 3-phosphate shuttle.

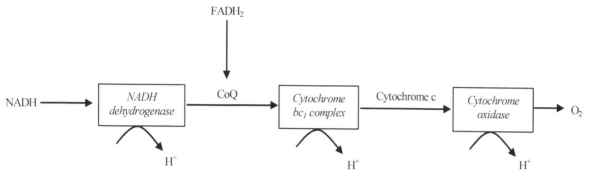

Figure 6.3 – Schematic of the electron transport chain

6.1.5.2 Reoxidation of reduced cofactors in the mitochondrion
As outlined above, the passage of reduced cofactors to the electron transport chain allows their reoxidation, and release of energy for creating a proton gradient.

NADH produced during glycolysis is located in the cytosol of the cell, whereas reoxidation can only occur in the mitochondrion. In addition, NADH is not able to freely diffuse across the mitochondrial membrane to be reoxidised. Thus, complex shuttle systems exist in which the 'reducing power' of NADH is transferred to a freely diffusible molecule, which can subsequently be reoxidised within the mitochondrion whilst reducing NAD^+ to NADH or FAD to $FADH_2$.

In most cells, the glycerol-3-phophate shuttle operates, with glycerol-3-phophate being the diffusible reduced molecule. In the heart and liver however, the more complex malate-aspartate shuttle, which uses activated transporters in the inner mitochondrial membrane to transfer malate, α-ketoglutarate, glutamate and aspartate into and out of the mitochondrion. Again this transfers 'reducing power' from the cytosol into the mitochondrial matrix.

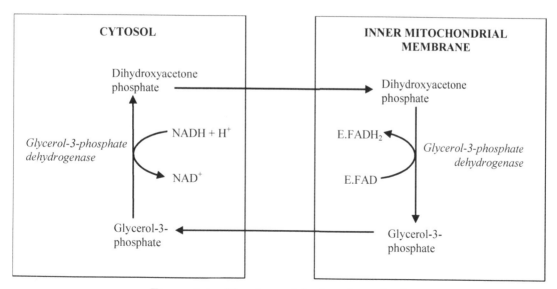

Figure 6.4 – The glycerol-3-phosphate shuttle

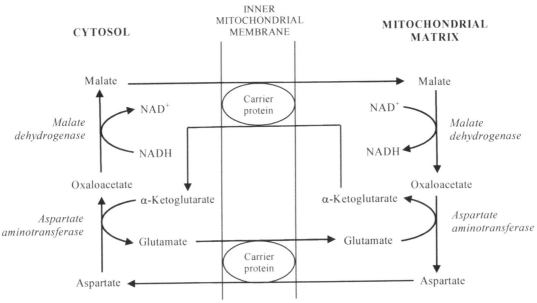

Figure 6.5 – The malate-aspartate shuttle

6.1.6 Mitochondrial ATP synthesis

6.1.6.1 The Chemiosmotic Mechanism

Oxidative phosphorylation describes the synthesis of ATP (i.e. phosphorylation of ADP or AMP) coupled to the oxidation of reduced cofactors NADH and $FADH_2$ by passage of electrons through the electron transport chain. It is distinguished from substrate level phosphorylation, which uses phosphorylated chemical intermediates create ATP.

The mechanism by which oxidation of reduced cofactors is coupled to the synthesis of ATP was proposed by Mitchell (1961), and is known as the chemiosmotic hypothesis. This states that the energy liberated by electron transport creates a proton gradient across the mitochondrial membrane, which may be used to synthesise ATP – thus, the proton gradient and not chemical intermediates are linked to ATP synthesis.

Chemiosmosis occurs in two broad stages – the creation of the proton gradient and the use of the energy stored in the gradient, with electrons flowing through membrane-bound ATP synthase.

Formation of the gradient

Along the electron transport chain, there is a fall in redox potential from one cofactor to another, thus releasing energy. The three main points of energy release are at the three main protein complexes – NADH dehydrogenase complex, cytochrome bc_1 complex and cytochrome oxidase complex. The energy released at these three stages is sufficient to pump protons from the matrix, across the inner mitochondrial membrane, and into the inter-membrane space.

Each of the protein complexes acts as the proton pump itself. Since $FADH_2$ only enters the electron transport chain after NADH dehydrogenase, its reoxidation is coupled only to two (and not three) sets of H^+ export.

Since protons are charged, the energy stored in the H^+ gradient across the inner mitochondrial membrane is related both to concentration and electrical potential. Thus, a very powerful electro-chemical proton gradient is formed, storing more energy than a simple chemical gradient using uncharged atoms.

Evidence for oxidation-linked gradient formation:
- Addition of a source of electrons (e.g. NADH) to a suspension of mitochondria depleted of oxygen results in no NADH oxidation.
- Addition of small amounts of O_2 to this suspension results in a sharp increase in the pH of the surrounding medium, corresponding to a decrease in the concentration of H^+ ions. This indicates movement of protons out of the matrix is coupled to the oxidation of NADH by O_2.
- Once O_2 has been depleted again, excess H^+ ions move back into the matrix, down the existing gradient, and thus the pH of the extracellular medium returns to normal.

Synthesis of ATP
Flow of protons back down their electrochemical gradient into the matrix, through ATP synthase drives ATP synthesis. Thus, ATP synthase is driven by proton-motive force (sum of electrical and chemical potential energy). It was originally believed 3 ATP molecules are synthesised per NADH, and 2 ATP per $FADH_2$. However, evidence now suggests these figures are more like 2.5 and 1.5, given the energy required for creating the proton gradient and various shuttle systems.

Evidence for ATP synthesis coupled to proton gradient usage
- Exposure of chloroplasts or mitochondria to an artificial proton gradient results in a burst of ATP synthesis, with the disappearance of the gradient.
- Oligomycin binds to the stalk of ATP synthase, blocking the central proton channel. This prevents re-entry of protons into the matrix meaning that pH and electrical gradients cannot the dissipated. Subsequently, the electron transport chain stops as complexes are working to pump against a steep gradient. This indicates electron transport and phospho-rylation are coupled processes – one cannot occur without the other.
- Uncoupling agents (e.g. 2,4-dinitrophenol, salicylic acid) act as H^+ ionophores to prevent ATP synthesis. These molecules carry protons across the inner mitochondrial membrane into the matrix, dissipating the gradient. The electron transport chain continues at an increased pace, but no electrochemical gradient is established and thus the energy is released as heat, rather than ATP (clinical application in treatment of obesity, although often results in death!).
- ATP is synthesised when reconstituted membrane vesicles containing bacteriorhodopsin (light driven proton pump that replaces the electron transport chain) and ATP synthase are illuminated. This shows the electron transport chain and ATP synthase are biochem-ically separate systems, linked only by the proton motive force.

6.1.6.2 Uses of the Proton Gradient

ATP synthesis
As outlined above, the proton gradient can be used in conjunction with ATP synthase to phosphor-ylate AMP or ADP to ATP. ATP synthase is an inner membrane enzyme complex through which protons flow back into the mitochondrial matrix. It consists of an F_1 subunit (site of ATP production) and an F_0 subunit (transmembrane pore through which ions flow). Around $3H^+$ pass through the pore for every ATP molecule synthesised.

The F_1 part contains 3α and 3β subunits resting on a γ subunit. ATP is synthesised spontaneously on the F_1 part of ATP synthase, even in the absence of a proton gradient, but ATP cannot leave the active site unless protons are flowing through the channel. Thus, the proton motive force passing through F_0 is required to release ATP.

Given the 3α and 3β subunits of F_1, which exist as αβ complexes, it is unsurprising that the enzyme cycles between three different states. Boyer's *Binding Change Mechanism* (1997 Nobel Prize) states the catalytic site (β subunit) rotates between these three states. In the open state (O), ADP and phosphate enter the active site. The protein then closes up around the molecules and binds them loosely – known as the loose state (L). The enzyme then undergoes another change in shape, catalysing ATP synthesis, with the active site in the resulting tight state (T) binding the newly-produced ATP molecule with very high affinity. Finally, the active site cycles back to the open state, releasing ATP and binding more ADP and phosphate, ready for the next cycle of ATP production. As such, at any one time one αβ complex is in O state, one in L state and one in T state. This means there is a constant production and release of ATP. In addition, the three sites show cooperativity – the binding of ADP and P_i to one site increases the release of ATP from another.

The changes in state described above are linked to the energy-requiring rotation of the γ subunit relative to the αβ parts. Evidence comes from F_1 complexes engineered to contain a β subunit adhered to a metal coated glass plate, with a γ subunit attached to a fluorescently labelled actin filament. Using fluorescent microscopy, actin filaments were seen to rotate in 120° steps in the presence of ATP, powered by the hydrolysis of ATP by β subunits – demonstrates rotation and that ATP synthase is a reversible enzyme and can be used to pump protons against their gradient.

Inner membrane transport
The proton motive force maybe also be used to transport substances in and out of the mitochondrion:
- ATP/ADP translocator – since most ATP is synthesised in the mitochondrion, yet used in the cytoplasm, it must be transported out. Similarly, ADP is most useful as a substrate within the mitochondrion, but most prevalent in the rest of the cell. Thus, energy from the H^+ electrochemical gradient is used to exchange these two molecules, bound to Mg. This uses around 25% of the proton gradient, explaining why 2.5 and 1.5 ATP are synthesised per NADH and $FADH_2$ respectively instead of 3 and 2.
- Various uptake proteins for substrates and ions e.g. Ca^{2+}, phosphate, pyruvate, citrate etc.

Thermogenesis in brown adipose tissue
Uncoupling of the proton motive force from ATP synthase results in the production of heat – called non-shivering thermogenesis. This is particular prevalent in brown adipose tissue, which contains many mitochondria. These possess the uncoupling protein thermogenin in their inner membrane, which allows the flow of protons back into the matrix, without passing through ATP synthase.

Brown adipose tissue is found in cold-exposed areas of newborn animals (including humans) and is important in maintaining temperature during hibernation.

6.1.7 Body Energy Supplies

Body stores:

Macromolecule	Weight (g)	Energy (Kcal)	Percentage of total
Fat	**10,000**	**90,000**	**74**
Carbohydrate (total)	**310**	**1240**	**2.8**
Liver glycogen	70	280	0.2
Muscle glycogen	225	900	0.75
Blood glucose	15	60	0.05
Protein (rare, requiring muscle breakdown)	**7,500**	**30,000**	**23**

Intake per day:

Macromolecule	Weight (g)	Energy (Kcal)
Fat	60	600
Carbohydrate	200	800
Protein	70	300

CHAPTER 7

Fat as a Metabolic Fuel

7.1 OVERVIEW

Fatty acid oxidation is central to body processes, since 35% of total energy is supplied by fats. In addition, many metabolic substrates can be converted to fats for efficient storage and fats provide important precursors for membrane synthesis, lipophilic modifiers of proteins, hormones and intracellular secondary messengers.

Advantages of fat metabolism
- Stores can be completely depleted without altering body function.
- Stores are dense – a large amount of energy is stored in a small volume. Also, large stores of fat are possible.
- Metabolism produces acetyl CoA directly, and the overall yield is very high (e.g. 129 ATP for palmitate) as fats are the most reduced form of carbon in the body.
- Rapid turnover is possible, which is ideal for tissues with high energy requirements.

Disadvantages of fat metabolism
- Some tissues, such as the brain, are unable to use fatty acids as substrates (although the brain can use ketone bodies, but these never reach high enough concentration to replace glucose as a fuel).
- Production of toxic ketoacids as by-products.
- Fats are highly insoluble in water, necessitating transport mechanisms.
- Nearly all animals are unable to convert fats to carbohydrates.

7.2 ASSIMILATION OF DIETARY FAT

Since dietary fat is insoluble in water, and unable to absorbed directly in the intestines, a sequence of events takes place to both absorb and transport fatty acids to where they are most needed. This involves various enzyme driven reactions, and relies on lipoproteins – globular, micelle-like particles

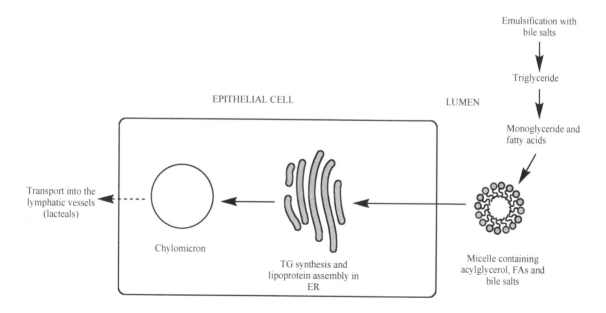

Figure 7.1 – Absorption of fats in the intestine

55

with a hydrophobic core of triacylglycerol and cholesterol esters, surrounded by an amphipathic coat of protein (called apolipoprotein), phospholipid and cholesterol.

7.2.1 Assimilation, emulsification and absorption
In the intestine, fat droplets from dietary intake of fatty foods are emulsified (forming a suspension of small globules of fat in the aqueous environment of the intestines) by bile salts from the liver. This reduces the size of the droplets, allowing lipolytic enzymes greater area to attack.

In the small intestine, lipases released from the pancreas digest the triglycerides in the fatty acids, forming monoglycerides and glycerol. These products are soluble enough to simply diffuse through the membrane of the brush border of the small intestine, without the need for active transporters.

7.2.2 Chylomicron synthesis, transport and uptake
Chylomicrons are the least dense and largest lipoproteins, containing small amounts of apolipoprotein A, B-48, C and E.

When monoglycerides and fatty acids are taken up by epithelial cells lining the small intestine, they are re-synthesised into triglycerides. These triglycerides are then packaged with apolipoproteins, cholesterol and phospholipids in the endoplasmic reticulum to form chylomicrons.

Chylomicrons are released from the lateral border of the epithelial cells at the level of nuclei by exocytosis into the local lymphatic system. In the intestine, the lymph vessels are know as lacteals, due to their milky colour from the presence of high amounts of fat. These have large enough fenestrations to allow chylomicrons through, unlike the mucosal capillaries which have an impenetrable basement membrane. Subsequently, the chylomicrons enter the systemic lymphatic system, passing into the subclavian vein and thus entering the blood stream.

In the blood, chylomicrons are acted on by lipoprotein lipases, releasing free fatty acids. These are taken up into the muscle and adipose tissue. Once all triglyceride have been depleted, the remaining chylomicron exists as a cholesterol-rich remnant which is taken up by the liver through receptor-mediated endocytosis.

7.2.3 Uptake, re-synthesis and use of triglyceride
The fatty acids released from the action of lipoprotein lipase can be taken up directly into cells. In adipose tissue, triglycerides are re-synthesised leading to the formation of fatty stores.

Triglyceride can also be used for energy, with breakdown through β-oxidation. This occurs in the skeletal muscle, heart and renal cortex. Note, fats are not used by the brain as an energy source.

7.2.4 NEFA – non-esterified fatty acids
Non-esterified fatty acids are merely those that are not bound to glycerol – i.e. are not part of a mono-, di- or triglyceride molecule. NEFAs are released from the lipolysis of stored triglyceride in adipose tissue, under the influence of hormone-sensitive lipase (HSL).

In the blood plasma, 99% of the free fatty acids are non-covalently bound to albumin. Albumin possesses at least 10 binding sites of which three are high affinity sites. This mechanism of transport is in contrast to triglycerides, which are too hydrophobic to be transported by albumin, and are therefore carried in lipoproteins. The main targets for NEFAs are the muscle, heart and liver. At these targets, the NEFAs are taken up passively, and bound to fatty acid binding protein within the cells. From here they may be used for energy or synthesis (especially liver).

The lipase used to free NEFAs from triglycerides is hormone controlled, allowing regulation of release of these high energy molecules:

Increase lipolysis	Decrease lipolysis
Adrenaline/Noradrenaline	Insulin
Glucagon	
TSH/T3	

As such, under different metabolic conditions the plasma level of NEFAs varies:

Condition	Plasma NEFA level (mmol/L)
Basal fed	0.3-0.6
Fasting overnight	0.5-2.0
Prolonged exercise	~2.0
Stress and trauma	0.8-1.8

These levels are low compared with glucose, but are relatively stable (in spite of rapid turnover) due to strong homeostatic functioning.

7.3 METABOLIC FUELS AND TISSUES
The three main tissues in the body that use triglycerides and NEFAs are the heart, skeletal muscle and renal cortex.

Heart
80% of the energy required for heart function comes from the β-oxidation of fatty acids. If this exogenous source is exhausted, the endogenous triglyceride stores are used, releasing NEFA. Generally, glucose is directed to glycogen synthesis in the heart, but can be used in extreme circumstances.

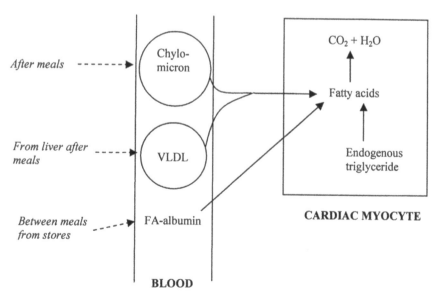

Figure 7.2 – Use of fatty acids in the heart

Skeletal Muscle

The use of NEFAs, glucose and glycogen in skeletal muscle varies depending on the type of fibres, and the length of exercise duration.

State	Plasma fatty acids/%	Plasma glucose/%	Intracellular glycogen/%
Rest	100	0	0
40 minutes exercise	37	27	36
90 minutes exercise	37	41	22
3 hours exercise	50	36	14
4 hours exercise	62	30	8

In general, slow fibres tend to use fatty acids more selectively whereas fast fibres are more glycolytic due to their rapid twitch activity.

Renal cortex

The renal cortex is highly energy demanding, due processes such as filtration. However, glucose upsets filtration gradients and therefore cannot be used as a metabolic substrate. The medulla, in contrast, has no blood supply and therefore is forced to use glucose due to the anaerobic conditions.

Energy source	Percentage usage
Fatty acids	>50
Endogenous triglycerides	40-50
Lactate and amino acids	5-10
Glucose	<1

7.4 OXIDATION OF FAT

The use of fatty acids for energy occurs with the sequential removal of two-carbon units from the chain (demonstrated by Knoop, correlating constituents of dog urine with the type of fatty acid they have been fed). The oxidation of fatty acids first requires their activation, with conversion to their acyl CoA derivative. Oxidation occurs in the mitochondrial matrix of eukaryotes and begins at the β-carbon of the chain, producing NADH, $FADH_2$ and acetyl CoA which may enter the electron transport chain and TCA cycle respectively.

There are three main steps in the oxidation of fatty acids:

7.4.1 Activation of fatty acids

Before entering the mitochondrial matrix, fatty acids are activated by the addition of CoA, to which it is bound via a thioester linkage. This reaction is catalysed by acyl CoA synthase (fatty acid thiokinase) present on the outer membrane of the mitochondrion, and requires one molecule of ATP. The product of this reaction is a fatty acyl CoA molecule.

7.4.2 Transport into mitochondria – the carnitine shuttle

Fatty acid chains up to 10 carbon atoms long are able to diffuse freely into mitochondria. However, those with longer chains are unable to do this, and therefore require a transport mechanism in which they are conjugated to carnitine. This transport occurs in a stepwise manner:
  1. Fatty acyl CoA conjugated to carnitine in exchange for the CoA group (using acyl carnitine acyltransferase I on the outer face of the inner mitochondrial membrane).
  2. Acyl carnitine is transported into the matrix using a translocase, in exchange for carnitine.

3. Once within the matrix, free carnitine is released and the CoA group is transferred back to the fatty acyl molecule using carnitine acyltransferase II on the matrix side of the inner mitochondrial membrane.

This is a key point of regulation in the degradation of fatty acids, through alteration of the activity of the carnitine-acylcarnitine translocase. This transporter is inhibited by malonyl CoA and thus, in the fasting state when there is decreased malonyl CoA, there is increased translocase activity and thus increased fatty acid oxidation. This occurs with a simultaneous increase in fatty acid release from stores by hormone-sensitive lipase during the fasting state.

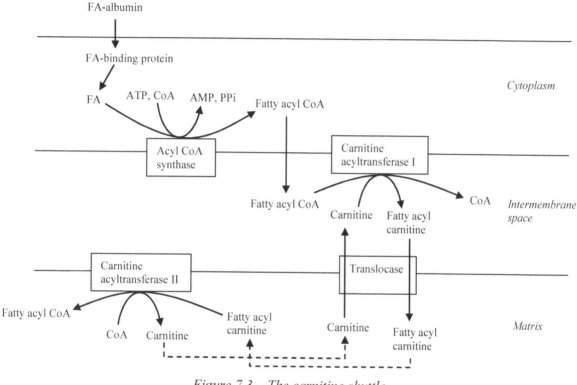

Figure 7.3 – The carnitine shuttle

Patients who have carnitine deficiency are unable to undergo efficient β-oxidation. This leads to cardiomyopathy (heart uses fatty acids), fatty infiltration of the organs (excess fatty acids deposited as unable to enter mitochondrion), skeletal muscle weakness and hypoglycaemia in 50% of cases. Treatment involves the administration of exogenous carnitine. This disease demonstrates the importance of fatty acid metabolism to the heart and skeletal muscle.

7.4.3 β-oxidation
β-oxidation of fatty acids occurs in four stages which repeat sequentially, releasing a two-carbon acetyl CoA molecule each time. These steps occur at the β-carbon of the chain – the third carbon along from the CoA end of the fatty acyl CoA molecule. The steps are:
1. Oxidation by acyl CoA dehydrogenase
2. Hydration by enoyl CoA hydratase
3. Oxidation by hydroxyacyl CoA dehydrogenase
4. Thiolysis by β-ketothiolase

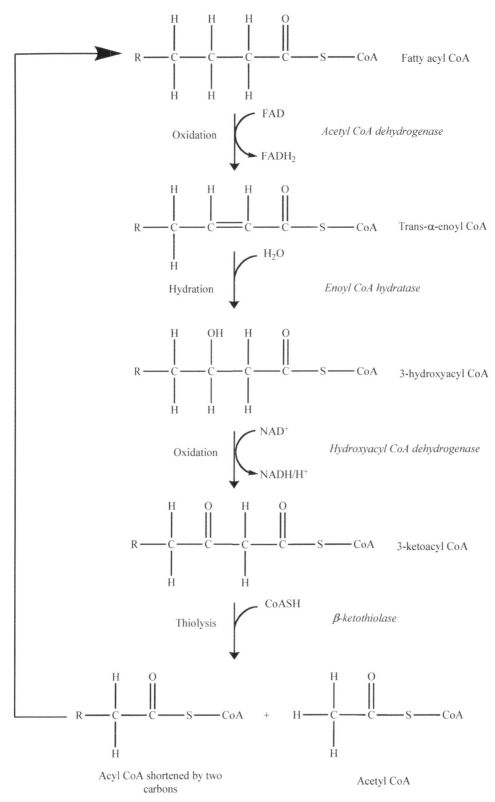

Figure 7.4 - β-oxidation of fatty acids

Sequential shortening of the fatty acid chain results in the release of two-carbon units. Eventually, a four-carbon molecule or five-carbon molecule (if originally odd-numbered fatty acid) is left, which is subsequently split into two molecules of acetyl CoA, or one acetyl CoA and one propionyl CoA.

Given the varying lengths of the fatty acid chains during this β-oxidation process, multiple fatty acyl CoA dehydrogenases (step 1) are needed, which are specific to acyl CoA molecules of different lengths:
- VLCAD – 20C to 14C
- LCAD – 18C to 12C
- MCAD – 14C to 12C
- SCAD – 6C to 4C

Note there is some overlap and gap left at each of the stages. The function of the enzymes is flexible (e.g. SCAD can operate on fatty acid chains of more than 6C sometimes), yet no single enzyme is able to catalyse all the reactions.

Clinical syndromes exist for deficiencies in each of these enzymes. For example, MCAD deficiency is present in 1 in 19,000 of the population, and shows infant onset. It causes a dramatic decrease in β-oxidation, leading to severe fasting hypoglycaemia (vomiting, lethargy, coma and death) with no ketosis during fasting as fatty acids can not be metabolised to ketones. It can be held responsible for 10% of cases of sudden infant death syndrome (SIDS).

The key mechanism of regulation of this stage of fatty acid metabolism is through the availability of substrate. Thus, breakdown of triglycerides by HSL into fatty acids in the liver is central to regulating the rate of β-oxidation. Thus, those hormones/conditions that increase and decrease the activity of HSL have an indirect impact on β-oxidation.

7.4.4 Oxidation of other fatty acids
Some fatty acids are unable to be degraded by the pathway described above, and therefore require specialised adaptations to allow the release of energy:

Unsaturated fatty acids with cis-bonds
- These are oxidised down to the 3-cis form by normal β-oxidation, and then converted to trans-fatty acids by an isomerase so β-oxidation can continue.

Very long chain fatty acids
- These are processed in peroxisomes and shortened to 16-18C chains, and then transferred to the mitochondrion for β-oxidation.
- Refsum's disease results from the specific peroxisomal enzyme deficiency, leading to the accumulation of very long chain fatty acids in the brain.

Odd chain fatty acids
- β-oxidation finishes with propionyl CoA, which is an important metabolic intermediate.

Branched chain fatty acids
- If the branch is present on the β-carbon then these fatty acids undergo α-oxidation instead, continuing normally and producing alternating acetyl CoA and propionyl CoA molecules.

7.4.4 Energy yield
Each cycle of β-oxidation (i.e. removal of one 2C unit) releases:
- 1 NADH (→ 3ATP)

- 1 FADH$_2$ ($\rightarrow$ 2ATP)
- 1 acetyl CoA ($\rightarrow$ 12 ATP through the TCA cycle)

Thus, there is a total yield of 17 ATP per round of β-oxidation, leading to a very high total yield for a single fatty acid molecule (e.g. 131 ATP for palmitoyl CoA).

7.5 FATTY ACID METABOLISM IN THE LIVER

7.5.1 Biosynthesis
In the fed state excess sugars and amino acids can be stored as triglyceride. This involves their conversion to fatty acid, and subsequent deposition in adipose tissue. This process occurs in the liver, and triglycerides are then moved to stores throughout the body in lipoproteins.

Fatty acid synthesis involves the condensation of two-carbon units (acetyl CoA) to form chains, but importantly it is not the reverse of β-oxidation (see later). There are three major stages:

Transport
Fatty acid synthesis occurs in the cytosol of hepatocytes, whilst the acetyl CoA produced from pyruvate and needed as a precursor for long fatty chains is present in the mitochondrion. Thus, a shuttle system is required to transport acetyl CoA into the cytosol.

Acetyl CoA is condensed with oxaloacetate in the mitochondrion to form citrate. This is then transported into the cytosol, where it is cleaved by ATP-citrate lysase to re-form oxaloacetate and acetyl CoA. Oxaloacetate is converted to malate and then pyruvate (producing NADPH), which may then pass back into the mitochondrion where it is carboxylated to oxaloacetate:

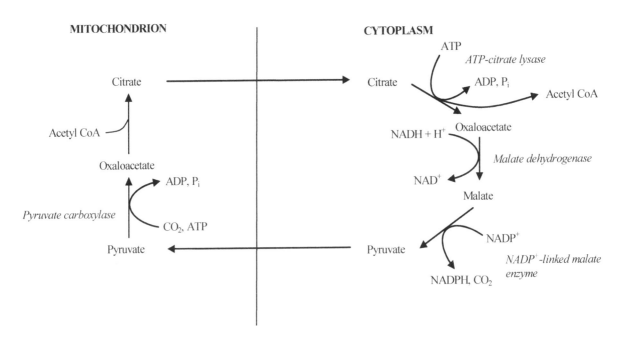

Figure 7.5 – The acetyl CoA shuttle

Carboxylation of acetyl CoA

The first committed step of fatty acid synthesis is the conversion of acetyl CoA into malonyl CoA by the addition of CO_2. This process is catalysed by acetyl CoA carboxylase, which is closely regulated and central to the control of fatty acid synthesis. This process uses one molecule of ATP.

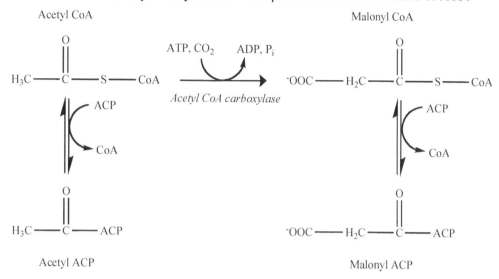

Figure 7.6 – Carboxylation of acetyl CoA

Regulation of acetyl CoA carboxylase operates by alternating between phosphorylated and dephosphorylated states. The enzyme is active when dephosphorylated, which occurs when energy levels are high, and substrates (i.e. acetyl CoA) plentiful:

	Activate	**Inhibit**
Covalent regulation	Dephosphorylated by protein phosphatase 2A - High ATP (inhibits kinase) - Insulin (activates phosphatase)	Phosphorylated by AMP-activated protein kinase - AMP (stimulates kinase) - Glucagon (inhibits phosphatase) - Adrenaline (inhibits phosphatase)
Allosteric regulation	Citrate (signal of high energy)	Palmitoyl CoA (high when abundant fatty acids)

Biosynthetic pathway

After the formation of malonyl CoA there are five steps in the creation and elongation of fatty acids:
1. Formation of acetyl and malonyl carrier proteins
2. Condensation of acetyl-ACP and malonyl-ACP
3. Reduction
4. Dehydration
5. Reduction

In order for elongation to occur, the intermediates must be linked to the phosphopantethine reactive unit present in acyl carrier proteins (ACP). Thus, the first step in the formation of fatty acids is the

63

synthesis of acetyl-ACP and malonyl-ACP from acetyl CoA and malonyl CoA. These reactions use acetyl transacylase and malonyl transacylase respective. Subsequently acetyl-ACP and malonyl-ACP are condensed together, creating a four-carbon chain which acts as the building block for elongation:

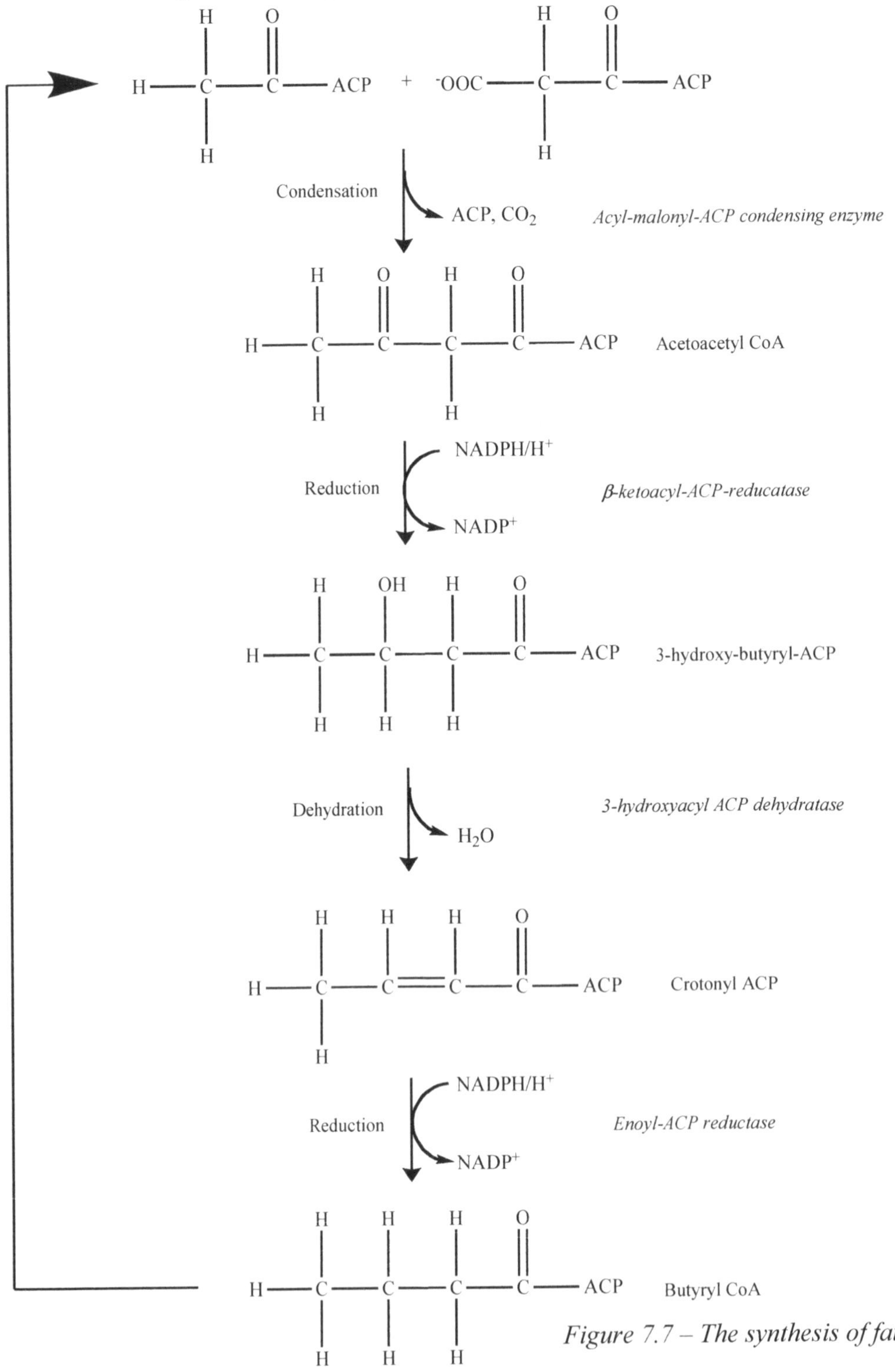

Figure 7.7 – The synthesis of fatty acids

The enzymes involved in the synthesis of fatty acids are all present in a single polypeptide chain as a multi-enzyme complex. This acts as a dimer, with each monomer having seven enzymatic domains. The arrangement increases the stability, coordination and efficiency of the reactions, with the flexible phosphopantethine unit of ACP carrying substrates between successive active sites. Per round of synthesis, 1 ATP (formation of malonyl ACP) and 2 NADPH molecules are used.

The process above is repeated, adding two-carbon malonyl CoA each time. This continues until 16C palmitoyl ACP is produced, which cannot the accepted by the condensing enzyme. Thus, a thioesterase releases palmitate and ACP, with subsequent elongation of palmitate taking place in the smooth endoplasmic reticulum using malonyl CoA rather than its ACP derivative.

Double bonds may be added to fatty acid chains up to C9. Therefore, certain fatty acids such as linoleic acid are essential since they cannot be synthesised, and must be obtained through the diet.

Long-term regulatory control occurs at the level of fatty acid synthesis. In addition to the acute regulation of acetyl CoA carboxylase, both this enzyme and fatty acid synthase adapt to prevailing conditions. Starvation prevents the synthesis of these enzymes, whilst an increase in insulin levels (in fed state) stimulates synthesis. Thus, animals fasted and then given a high carbohydrate, low fat diet show marked increases in the levels of these enzymes.

Synthesis of triglycerides
The final stage in the storage of energy as fats is the synthesis of triglyceride in adipose tissue. Fatty acids created in the above reaction are esterified to glycerol to form storable lipid .

Comparison of fatty acid synthesis and degradation
In order to prevent futile cycling (when two metabolic pathways run simultaneously in opposite directions, having no overall effect other than wasting energy), the degradation and synthesis of fatty acids are not reverse pathways. Indeed, they show many marked differences.

	Synthesis	Degradation
Subcellular location	Cytosol (liver only)	Mitochondrial matrix (muscle and liver)
Carriers between mitochondria and cytosol	Citrate	Carnitine
Phophopantetheine containing unit	ACP	CoA
Redox cofactor	NADPH	NAD^+ and FAD
Enzymes	Single, multienzyme complex	Discrete enzymes
Key regulatory point	Acetyl CoA carboxylase	Carnitine transporter, HSL
Activator	Citrate	
Inhibitor	Fatty acyl CoA	Malonyl CoA
Hormonal state favouring pathway	High insulin:glucagon ratio	Low insulin:glucagon ratio
Product	Palmitoyl CoA	Acetyl CoA

7.5.2 Ketogenesis
During prolonged fasting, the rates of β-oxidation and production of acetyl CoA increase due to release of fatty acids from lipid stores. However, the amount of acetyl CoA produced often exceeds

the amount required for entry into the TCA cycle, and thus excess acetyl CoA is converted into ketones. This occurs in the liver, in what is effectively a reverse of the thiolysis step of β-oxidation:

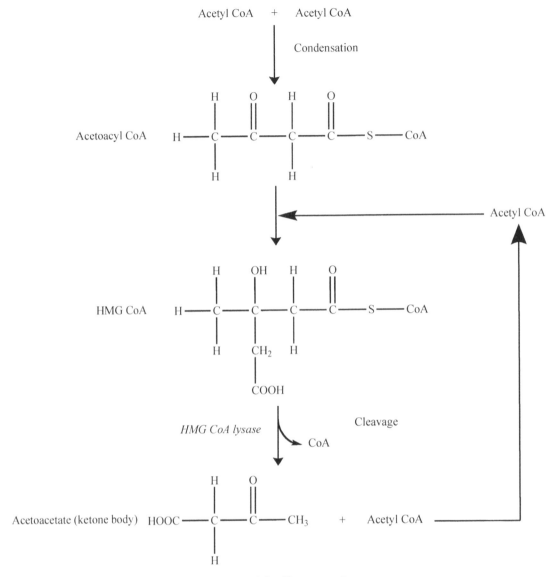

Figure 7.8 - Ketogenesis

Ketones (e.g. acetoacetate, acetone, 3-hydroxybutyrate) are water soluble molecules which can be used as a preferential substrate by heart muscle and renal cortex during fasting. In addition, they can be used by the brain during prolonged fasting and thus provide an important alternative when glucose is unavailable. They are easily activated and metabolised, and their usage restricts the depletion of limited glucose stores. The oxidation of ketones in peripheral tissues occurs in proportion to their plasma concentration. When given with fatty acids and glucose, they are the preferred substrate, suggesting ketone oxidation suppresses the usage of these other fuels:

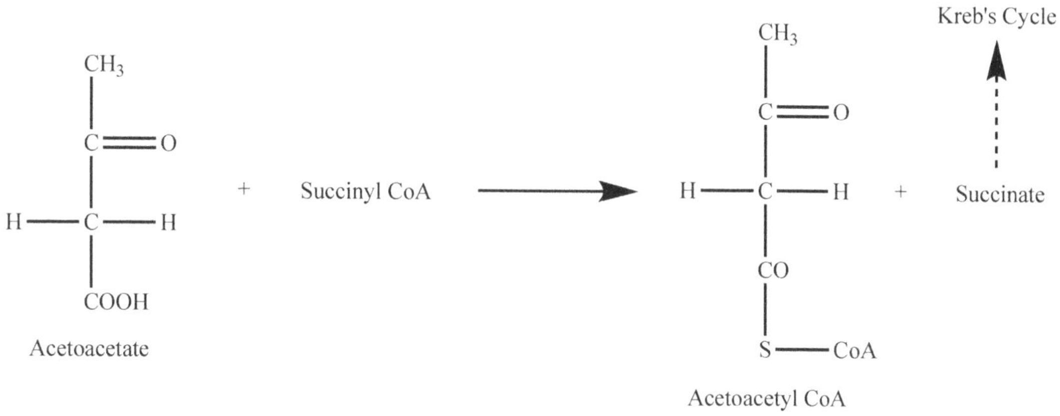

$$CH_3 - C(=O) - CH(H)(COOH) \quad \text{(Acetoacetate)} \quad + \quad \text{Succinyl CoA} \quad \longrightarrow \quad CH_3 - C(=O) - CH_2 - CO - S - CoA \quad \text{(Acetoacetyl CoA)} \quad + \quad \text{Succinate} \rightarrow \text{Kreb's Cycle}$$

Figure 7.9 – Ketone oxidation

The plasma concentration of glucose rises rapidly after one day's fasting, and much earlier than this in children. They are used by the kidney, skeletal muscle, heart muscle and the brain (after 48 hours). In addition, foetuses are able to use ketones, which also inhibit the use of glucose, lactate and amino acids needed for development. Thus, during pregnancy the maternal levels of plasma ketones increases, allowing them to cross the placenta where they can act as an energy substrate and lipogenic precursor.

Ketone bodies act as signals for the availability of energy substrates. Thus, high levels indicating a fasting state increase the rate of gluconeogenesis and prevent the storage of metabolic molecules.

In diabetes, acetoacetate is produced faster than it can be metabolised by peripheral tissues (diabetes can be described as 'fasting in the face of plenty'). Thus, untreated diabetics often have high levels of ketone bodies in their blood, leading to characteristic 'acetone breath' which smells like pear drops.

7.6 INTEGRATION OF FATTY ACID METABOLISM

Insulin – the fed state

Increase	Decrease
Lipoprotein lipase activity, clearing of chylomicrons	Mobilisation of free fatty acids from adipose tissue
Uptake of glucose by adipose tissue by GLUT4 → glycerol and triglyceride synthesis	
Pentose phosphate pathway to generate NADPH (for fatty acid synthesis)	
Synthesis of fatty acid synthase and acetyl CoA carboxylase	

67

Glucagon – the fasting state

Increase	Decrease
Hormone sensitive lipase activity, releasing free fatty acids from adipose tissue	Acetyl CoA carboxylase activity
	Synthesis of fatty acid synthase and acetyl CoA carboxylase

Adrenaline – the fasting state

Increase	Decrease
Hormone sensitive lipase activity, releasing free fatty acids from adipose tissue	Acetyl CoA carboxylase activity
	Synthesis of fatty acid synthase and acetyl CoA carboxylase

Thyroxine – the fasting state

Increase	Decrease
Acyl CoA-carnitine acyltransferase activity increasing uptake into mitochondria	Fatty acid synthesis
Ketogenesis	Secretion of lipoproteins (with increased clearance)
Adipose tissue lipolysis	

In the hyperthyroid state (high thyroxine) fatty acid oxidation and ketogenesis are stimulated simultaneously with a paradoxical stimulation of fatty acid synthesis. Esterification of fatty acid to triglyceride is reduced, as is the secretion of VLDL. In the intact animal or patient, however, serum triglyceride concentration is variable, which may reflect increased adipose tissue lipolysis and elevated concentrations of plasma FFA, which would tend to drive VLDL secretion by the liver.

Clearance of VLDL and LDL is increased in high thyroxine levels, resulting in decreased plasma total cholesterol and LDL cholesterol. Although HDL cholesterol may also be reduced, the ratio of LDL:HDL cholesterol is further decreased.

In the hypothyroid, many of these effects are reversed, which results in hyperlipoproteinemias and greater risk for the development of atherosclerotic cardiovascular disease.

CHAPTER 8

Glucose as a Metabolic Fuel

8.1 OVERVIEW

Glucose is a very important energy source, particularly for the brain and red blood cells, which rely almost exclusively on glucose under normal conditions. Glucose comes from dietary intake, glycogen stores and synthesis from other biochemical compounds.

Stores
Generally available – 70g in liver and kidney
Local usage – 220g in muscle

Liver stores are sufficient to provide the brain with glucose for about 12 hours during fasting. Thus, during periods of fasting and vigorous exercise, gluconeogenesis is required to maintain blood glucose levels.

Intake
Glucose – 100g per day
Fructose – 100g per day

Usage
Aerobic – 110g per day by the brain
Anaerobic – 25g per day by red blood cells, 30g per day by renal medulla, 30g per day by skeletal muscle
Total – 195g per day

8.2 GLYCOLYSIS

8.2.1 Significance

Glycolysis occurs in the cytoplasm of cells. The overall scheme involves the conversion of glucose to pyruvate via a series of reactions, generating energy (directly and via pyruvate conversion to acetyl CoA, which may enter TCA cycle) and providing many important intermediates for biosynthesis.

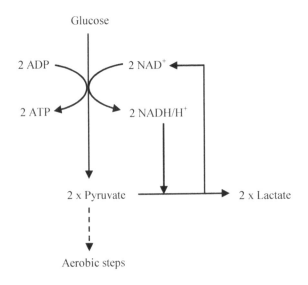

Figure 8.1 – Overview of glycolysis

Glycolysis is essential since it provides the only way to generate ATP under anaerobic conditions. Thus, partial oxidation of glucose to lactate in cells unable to metabolise aerobically (erythrocytes, renal medulla, lens of eye, muscle during prolonged exercise) can obtain 2 ATP per glucose molecule, which represents around 1/20 of the maximum yield possible.

Glycolysis is therefore necessary when:
- Supply of oxygen can not keep up with usage (strenuous exercise).
- Supply of oxygen fails (hypoxia, ischaemia).
- Cells are unable to metabolise aerobically (erythrocytes have no mitochondria, renal medulla has poor blood flow and oxygen provision).

8.2.2 Glucose uptake (transport and phosphorylation)

Glucose uptake is a complex process, designed to meet the different roles of glucose in various cells around the body. It is achieved mainly by the transporters GLUT 1, 2, 3, 4, 5 and 7. Each of these has a specific distribution and set of kinetic properties.

Transporter	Location	Properties and role
GLUT 1 and 3	Nearly all mammalian cells – widely distributed	- Responsible for constant basal glucose uptake. - K_m is 1mM whereas blood glucose concentration is 5mM, leading to constant transport rate not affected by [glucose]. - Uptake depends on energy needs of the cell.
GLUT 2	Liver, pancreatic β-cells, intestine (glucose absorption)	- Very high K_m of 15-20mM (i.e. low affinity). - Uptake of glucose into tissues proportional to the [glucose] in the surrounding environment, allowing it to act as a sensor of glucose concentration: ▪ Liver glycogen and fat synthesis. ▪ Pancreatic hormone production. - Allows glucose to enter vital organs such as the brain when [glucose] low, since unable to compete with GLUT 1 and 3 in affinity for substrate.
GLUT 4	Muscle, adipose tissue	- Insulin responsive, allowing increased glucose uptake after meals for energy/storage in adipose tissue. - After meals, more transporters fuse with plasma membrane in insulin signal-dependent manner.
GLUT 5	Small intestine	- Uptake and concentration of dietary fructose. - Works in tandem with glucose/Na^+ symporter.
GLUT 7	Endoplasmic reticulum	

Phosphorylation

Once glucose has entered cells, it is necessary to 'trap' it there, preventing it from diffusing out down its concentration gradient. This is done by the first reaction of glycolysis – phosphorylation of glucose to glucose-6-phosphate – which also activates the substrate. In addition to trapping glucose, this process allows more glucose to diffuse into the cell through simple transporters as glucose-6-phosphate does not affect the glucose concentration gradient.

$$Glucose + ATP \rightarrow Glucose\text{-}6\text{-}phophate + ADP$$

This process is performed by two enzymes:
-   Hexokinase – present in all peripheral tissues. Has a high affinity for glucose and is inhibited by glucose-6-phosphate.
-   Glucokinase – present in the liver and pancreatic β-cells, working along side GLUT 2. It has a low affinity for glucose, and thus acts as a sensor, forming glucose-6-phophate in a concentration-dependent manner and only when [glucose] is high. This is the initial (and controlled) step in glycogenesis. Glucokinase can not metabolise fructose.

8.2.3 Trapping energy: formation of ATP in glycolysis

Glycolysis is a series of reactions taking place in the cytoplasm of cells. Overall, it involves the conversion of one molecule of glucose into two molecules of pyruvate. In doing so, 4 ATP molecules are generated, although two are used in the early steps of the glycolytic pathway. This leads to a net yield of 2 ATP per glucose molecule.

These ATP molecules are generated by substrate-level phosphorylation – the formation of ATP by the direct transfer of a phosphate group to ADP from a reactive intermediate, occurring under both aerobic and anaerobic conditions. Unlike oxidative phosphorylation (which generates the majority of ATP form glucose by feeding acetyl CoA into the TCA cycle), here oxidation and phosphorylation are not coupled.

ATP formation occurs at the conversion of 1,3-bisphosphoglycerate to 3-phosphoglycerate by phosphoglycerate kinase and the conversion of phosphoenolpyruvate to pyruvate by pyruvate kinase.

8.2.4 Control of glycolysis

Glycolysis, being a key pathway in the generation of energy and usage of an important metabolic substrate, is tightly controlled in response to the energy needs of the cells. Given the varying requirements of different tissues in the body, this regulation varies from cell to cell:
-   Brain – no control since there is a steady high-flow rate through glycolysis to pyruvate, in order to feed the TCA cycle for complete oxidation in the mitochondria. This is reflected in the brain's selective usage of glucose.
-   Muscle – acute and rapid alteration in the glycolytic pathway since the high energy demand of this tissue is only met by anaerobic glycolysis. This is particularly important in type IIb muscle (fast-glycolytic) fibres which are the fastest firing and most powerful, twitching at upwards of 120 times per second. These fibres have a low oxidative demand, with a lack of myoglobin and mitochondria (relative to the Type I and Type IIa fibres) and thus rely exclusively on anaerobic energy production.

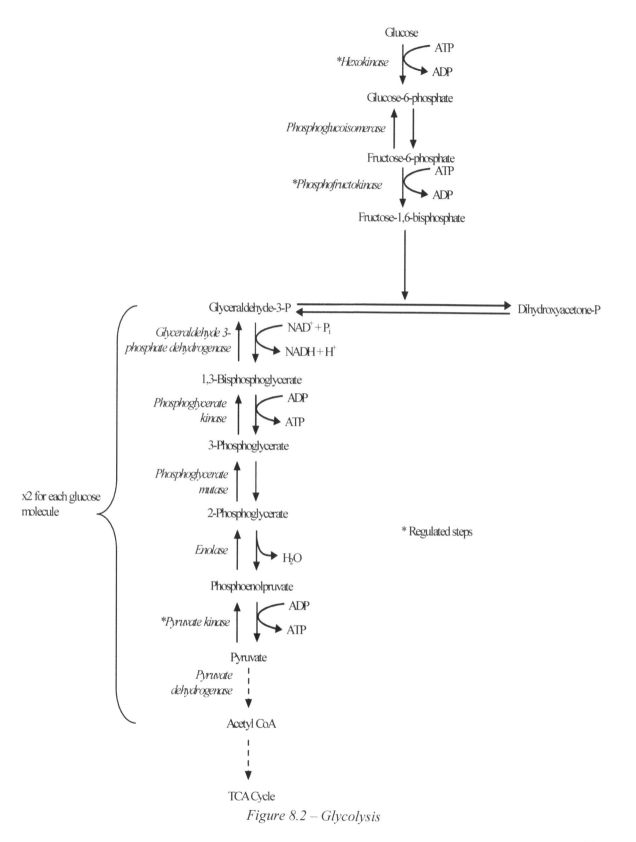

Figure 8.2 – Glycolysis

Points of regulation in all metabolic pathways are always irreversible reactions, and often operate far from equilibrium. This makes them committed steps. In glycolysis, the reactions of this type are catalysed by three enzymes:
- Hexokinase
- Phosphofructokinase
- Pyruvate kinase

8.2.4.1 Hexokinase
Hexokinase catalyses the formation of glucose-6-phosphate from glucose (using one ATP molecule). This is the first irreversible step of glycolysis, but unusually it is not the most important in control despite being the first step. This is because glucose-6-phosphate also feeds into glycogen synthesis and the pentose phosphate pathway, and thus this is not the first step *unique* to glycolysis.

Inhibit   **Activate**

Glucose-6-phosphate

The inhibition of hexokinase by glucose-6-phosphate is important in the control of phosphofructokinase as well. Inhibition of PFK by its own regulators (see below) leads to a build up of fructose-6-phosphate and thus a build up of glucose-6-phophate. This in turn inhibits hexokinase, which prevents the initial step of glycolysis and thus inhibits PFK further by not providing it with any substrate. This makes the PFK catalysed step the most important in control.

8.2.4.2 Phosphofructokinase
Phosphofructokinase catalyses the conversion of fructose-6-phosphate to fructose-1,6-bisphosphate, again using one molecule of ATP. This is the most important regulatory step in glycolysis.

Inhibit

ATP – allosteric inhibition, reducing affinity for fructose-6-phosphate.

Citrate – first product of the TCA cycle, and therefore signals there is a plentiful supply of intermediates for the cycle. Thus, no additional glycolysis is needed.

H^+ ions – slows down glycolysis when pH is low. Prevents the formation of excessive lactic acid, and thus acidosis when high levels of anaerobic respiration.

Activate

AMP – reverses the effect of ATP, allowing the enzyme to be responsive to cell energy levels.

Fructose-2,6-bisphosphate – strongly activates PFK. Synthesised from fructose-6-phosphate, signalling a high level of substrate for PFK and thus suitable conditions for rapid glycolysis.

Fructose-2,6-bisphosphate (Note: not fructose-**1,6**-bisphosphate) is an important molecule in the regulation of PFK. It is synthesised from fructose-6-phosphate by phosphofructokinase 2, with the reverse reaction catalysed by fructose bisphosphatase 2. These two enzymes are on the same bifunctional polypeptide.

74

Fructose-6-phophate regulates the formation of fructose-2,6-bisphosphate by activating the kinase whilst inhibiting the phosphatase. In addition, the bifunctional enzyme is also sensitive to phosphorylation, allowing control by glucagon and insulin and thus regulation of glycolysis by these hormones:

Signal molecule	Effect on phosphofructokinase 2	Effect on fructose bisphosphatase 2	Effect on fructose-2,6-bisphosphate and PFK
Fructose-6-phosphate	Activate	Inhibit	Increase Activate enzyme
Insulin – cAMP dependent dephosphorylation of bifunctional enzyme	Activate	Inhibit	Increase Activate enzyme
Glucagon – cAMP dependent phosphorylation of bifunctional enzyme	Inhibit	Activate	Lower Inhibit enzyme

8.2.4.3 Pyruvate kinase
Pyruvate kinase is responsible for the formation of pyruvate from phosphoenolpyruvate. This is the final step before the formation of acetyl CoA, and thus feeding into the TCA cycle. In addition, pyruvate is a key point for the generation of other products such as lactate and ethanol.

Inhibit	Activate
ATP – high energy levels so none needed from TCA cycle.	Fructose-1,6-bisphosphate – feed-forward control.
Alanine – signals levels of biosynthetic precursors, none needed from TCA cycle.	
Glucagon – via cAMP dependent phosphorylation.	

8.2.4.4 Isoenzymes
Glycolysis uses two enzymes which are present in isoenzyme form – lactate dehydrogenase and pyruvate kinase. Isoenzymes are different forms of the same enzyme, possessing varying kinetic properties. Different isoenzymes are expressed selectively in certain tissues, allowing tailoring to specific metabolic functions.

Lactate dehydrogenase
- Catalyses the interconversion of lactate and pyruvate.
- Exists as a tetramer of two subunits – H (mainly in heart) and M (mainly in muscle and liver).

- Five different forms exist – H_4, H_3M_1, H_2M_2, H_1M_3 and M_4 in order of affinity for substrate. In addition, H_4 is strongly inhibited by pyruvate, whilst it has sequentially decreasing effect on the other isoenzymes with M_4 not being affected by pyruvate at all.
- Role in heart – conversion of lactate to pyruvate for energy.
- Role in liver – conversion of lactate to pyruvate, and subsequently to glucose for gluconeogenesis.
- Role in muscle – conversion of pyruvate to lactate for maintaining glycolysis and purging of pyruvate.

Pyruvate kinase
- Catalyses formation of pyruvate from phosphoenolpyruvate.
- Also present in tetrameric form – M (mainly muscle for contraction and brain) and L (liver).
- Major difference between the subunits that make up the enzymes is their ability to be regulated, with only the L-form being affected via glucagon-dependent phosphorylation, decreasing the activity of the enzyme
  - Reflects the different roles of the enzyme in the different tissues.
  - Highly important that gluconeogenesis only occurs in low glucose conditions – must inhibit enzyme involved in the breakdown of glucose.
  - Muscle contraction only requires ATP from glycolysis, so regulation is much less important – merely dependent on need.

Isoenzymes are clinically important, since detection of a specific subset in blood tests can indicate localised tissue damage.

8.2.5 Utilisation of other monosaccharides
The human diet provides many non-glucose monosaccharides which are also able to provide energy. These include galactose and fructose.

Galactose
Lactose, present in milk, is a major source of carbohydrate in babies. Hydrolysis of this disaccharide yields glucose and galactose. Galactose is converted to glucose in order to be used:

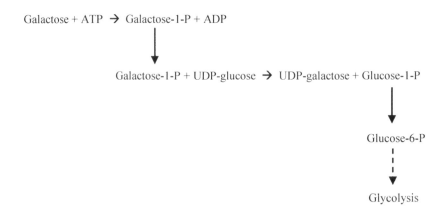

Galactose + ATP → Galactose-1-P + ADP

Galactose-1-P + UDP-glucose → UDP-galactose + Glucose-1-P

Glucose-6-P

Glycolysis

Figure 8.3 – Conversion of galactose to glucose

Inability to convert galactose to glucose can result in a build up of toxic compounds. This is known as galactosaemia. First milk ingestion in babies with this disease results in vomiting, severe liver disease and a failure to thrive. The only treatment is the restriction of galactose from the diet, although complications such as mental retardation still occur.

Fructose
Fructose intake is high in the Western diet, with sources including table sugar (sucrose, which is hydrolysed to glucose and fructose), fruits and honey. There are two pathways for fructose metabolism, one occurring in the muscle and adipose tissue and the other occurring in the liver.

Muscle and adipose – fructose phosphorylated by hexokinase, forming fructose-6-phosphate, which may enter glycolysis.

Liver – liver only possesses glucokinase, and therefore cannot phosphorylate fructose. Thus, fructokinase converts fructose to fructose-1-phosphate, which is then split into glyceraldehyde and dihydroxyacetone phosphate by fructose-1-phosphate aldolase. Dihydroxyacetone phosphate enters glycolysis directly at the triose phosphate isomerase step, whilst glyceraldehyde is first converted to glyceraldehyde-3-phosphate by triose kinase, and can then feed into glycolysis:

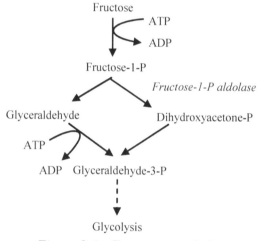

Figure 8.4 – Fructose metabolism

This process is unregulated, since the substrates enter glycolysis below the controlled step.

In hereditary fructose intolerance there is a defect in frustose-1-phosphate aldolase. This results in sweating, trembling, dizziness, nausea and vomiting on fructose ingestion. In addition, it can lead to hypoglycaemia and hypophosphataemia with an increase in lactate, alanine, glucose and fatty acids.

8.3 AEROBIC OXIDATION OF GLUCOSE

8.3.1 Entry into the TCA cycle
Glycolysis releases very little energy in itself, and therefore under aerobic conditions pyruvate is converted to acetyl CoA in the mitochondrial matrix such that it may be fed into the TCA cycle. The TCA cycle is capable of generating considerable amounts of reduced co-factors, and thus generating ATP via the electron transport chain.

The conversion of pyruvate to acetyl CoA is carried out by pyruvate dehydrogenase. This enzyme controls the balance between the usage of different energy substrates under varying conditions, and is therefore closely regulated in response to metabolic status in the mitochondrion.

Pyruvate dehydrogenase is a large multi-enzyme complex consisting of 210 subunits. It is regulated by phosphorylation, with the dephosphorylated state being more active. Interconversion between the two states is under the control of PDH kinase and PDH phosphatase. The enzymes are in turn allosterically regulated by energy levels. Pyruvate dehydrogenase is inactive when metabolic activity in the mitochondrion reflects an abundance of substrate (i.e. high ATP, acetyl CoA and NADH):

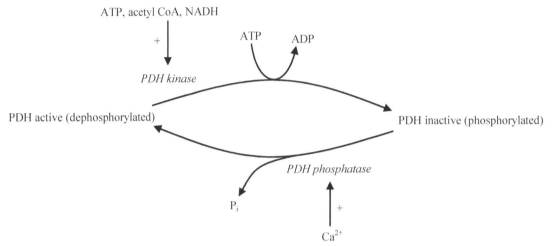

Figure 8.5 – Regulation of pyruvate dehydrogenase

The aerobic oxidation of glucose is particularly important in the brain since energy can not be obtained from fatty acids or other substrates. Ketogenesis in the brain results in neurological impairment.

8.3.2 Pentose phosphate pathway
In the cell, reducing power for various metabolic reactions comes from NADH and NADPH, amongst other reduced co-factors. In general, NADH is used for ATP production, whilst NADPH is important in biosynthesis. Unfortunately, these two co-factors are not interchangeable, and therefore reactions are needed to synthesise NADPH. The pentose phosphate pathway is responsible for the synthesis of NADPH. In addition, it is able to interconvert sugar phosphates, including pentoses, which are essential for the formation of nucleic acids.

The pentose phosphate pathway is particularly important in tissues that synthesise fatty acids and steroids from acetyl CoA, such as adipose tissue, the mammary glands and adrenal cortex. It occurs in the cytosol of cells.

The pathway occurs in three broad steps:
1. Irreversible oxidation of glucose-6-phosphate to 6-phosphoglucuronic acid and then ribulose-5-phosphate, generating two NADPH molecules.

2. Isomerisation of ribulose-5-phosphate to ribose-5-phosphate which may be used in nucleic acid synthesis.
3. Linkage of pentose phosphate pathway to glycolysis (when ribose-5-phosphate not needed for synthesis) via the irreversible interconversion of sugar phosphates using transketolase and transaldolase.

Control of the pentose phosphate pathway is afforded by the inhibition of glucose-6-phosphate dehydrogenase by NADPH, and activation by $NADP^+$.

The pentose phosphate pathway is also important in removal of oxidants, as shown by glucose-6-phosphate dehydrogenase deficiency (favism). This is a very common disease in which patients develop acute haemolytic anaemia on ingestion of oxidant drugs (e.g. antibiotics, antimalarials and antipyretics) or other compounds (e.g. fava beans). NADPH is used to generate reduced glutathione from glutathione. Reduced glutathione is then used to reduce H_2O_2 (a highly dangerous oxidising agent), being oxidised in the process. Thus, without the pentose phosphate pathway and generation of NADPH, H_2O_2 accumulates in cells and causes erythrocyte membrane rupture.

8.4 STORAGE OF GLUCOSE

8.4.1 Glycogen metabolism
In animal cells, excess glucose can be stored as glycogen. Glycogen is a very large, highly hydrated branching polymer of glucose which occupies a large volume in the cell. The fact that glycogen is relatively non-dense compared to other stored macromolecules (e.g. triglyceride) means storage is limited, and glycogen only represents 1% of the total body energy stores.

Glycogen is present in almost all tissues of the body, but particularly in the liver (as granules in the cytosol) and muscles. In the liver, it helps to maintain constant blood glucose levels, whilst in the muscle glycogen provides a local source of glucose for contraction.

The synthesis and breakdown of glycogen occur via two separate pathways which are reciprocally regulated in order to prevent futile cycling. Regulation occurs principally from allosteric and hormonal control.

8.4.1.1 Glycogen synthesis
The synthesis of glycogen utilises a derivative of glucose called UDP-glucose, and occurs in three enzymatic steps:

1. Conversion of glucose-6-phosphate to glucose-1-phosphate by glucose isomerase, and then the conversion of glucose-1-phosphate to UDP-glucose (using one UTP) catalysed by UDP-glucose pyrophosphorylase.
2. Addition of UDP-glucose to existing $(glycogen)_n$ chain, forming $(glycogen)_{n+1}$ and releasing UDP. Catalysed by glycogen synthase at non-reducing end of glycogen chain, forming an α-1,4-glycosidic link.
3. Insertion of branches into the chain via transglycosylase enzyme. This enzyme removes one end from the chain by hydrolysing an α-1,4-glycosidic link, and reattaches it via an α-1,6-glycosidic link.

Glycogen synthase is only able to extend an existing glycogen chain. Therefore, an initial primer, glycogenin, is needed. This primer consists of a small protein with eight glucose residues attached, to which additional UDP-glucose may be added. Importantly, glycogen synthase is only active when in contact with glycogenin which therefore limits the size of granules since only one primer is present in each granule.

Glycogen synthase is not able to insert branches into the chain, hence the need for the transglycosylase enzyme. Branches in the polymer increase its solubility and increase the rate of eventual hydrolysis since more exposed ends are present for degradation enzymes to operate on.

Overall, it costs 1 ATP molecule per glucose monomer added to the glycogen chain due to the need to form UTP which can be used in the synthesis of UDP-glucose.

8.4.1.2 Glycogen degradation
The mobilisation of glycogen is not a direct reversal of glycogen synthesis. This is because the thermodynamics of breakdown do not permit synthesis at physiological ratios, and the hormones that increase breakdown inhibit synthesis. This is demonstrated by patients with McArdles disease, who lack muscle glycogen phosphorylase. Thus, they are able to synthesise glycogen, but not break it down leading to large glycogen deposits in the muscles and stiffness during exercise.

The breakdown of glycogen requires three enzymes:

1. Glycogen phosphorylase – catalyses the phosphorolysis (uses inorganic phosphate) of α-1,4-glycosidic links, releasing glucose-1-phosphate.
2. Transferase – glycogen phosphorylase is unable to remove glucose monomers up to four before a branch point, therefore two enzymes are used to overcome this problem. Transferase removes all but the first glucose from a branch, and attaches them to the end of the unbranched chain by α-1,4-glycosidic links.
3. Debranching enzyme – acts as an α-1,6-glucosidase, removing the final glucose monomer to which the branch was originally attached. Thus, a branched molecule is converted into a linear one, allowing glycogen phosphorylase to continue as normal.

The product of glycogen breakdown is glucose-1-phosphate. This is converted by a mutase enzyme into glucose-6-phosphate for use in the liver and muscle:
- Liver – glucose-6-phosphatase converts glucose-6-phosphate into glucose, which is then able to enter the bloodstream
- Muscle – no glucose-6-phosphatase present, so glucose-6-phosphate merely passes straight into glycolysis for the generation of energy.

8.4.2 Control of glycogen metabolism
The metabolism of glycogen must be closely regulated to ensure energy is released when demand is high, and stored when glucose is abundant. In addition, reciprocal regulation of the synthase and phosphorylase enzymes ensure futile cycling of substrate molecules and wasteful hydrolysis of UTP are prevented. Regulation occurs through covalent modification, allosteric control and hormonal regulation.

8.4.2.1 Regulation of glycogen synthase
Glycogen synthase is regulated by phosphorylation and allosteric effects. Substrates and hormones can affect the relative activities of protein phosphatase I and protein kinase A, allowing a shift in phosphorylation state. However, to become fully active, additional allosteric effects are also required:

The shift between glycogen synthase a and b under the influence of the kinase and phosphatase is operating over the *chronic* timescale. However, note that inactive glycogen synthase b can be

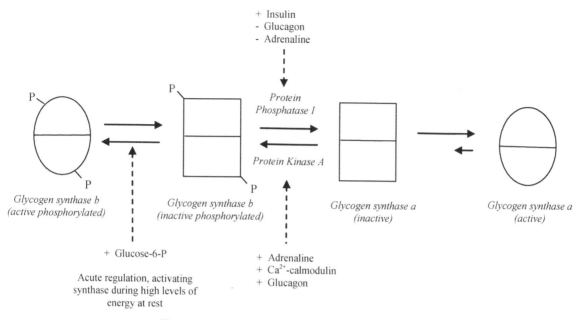

Figure 8.6 – Regulation of glycogen synthase

activated *acutely* through an increase in glucose-6-phosphate level. This requires very high levels of substrate, and therefore only occurs at rest. Glycogen synthase a, however, is under no such allosteric control and is therefore effectively only transiently inactive.

Overall, glycogen synthase is active when there are signals of high energy and substrate level, whilst inactive when glucose and energy levels are low, necessitating glycogen breakdown.

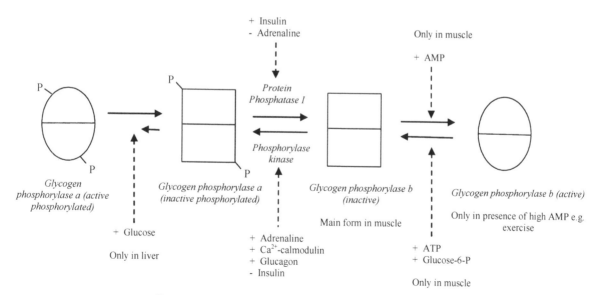

Figure 8-7 – Regulation of glycogen phosphorylase

8.4.2.2 Regulation of glycogen phosphorylase

Glycogen phosphorylase is also regulated by phosphorylation and allosteric control. In general, anything that stimulates the synthase enzyme will inhibit the phosphorylase enzyme. Thus, overall the phosphorylase is active when levels of glucose are low and inactive when blood glucose concentrations are high. This emphasises the importance of insulin and glucagon in their control.

Note, differences exist between the regulation in the muscle and liver in glycogen phosphorylase. Glycogen phosphorylase exists mainly in the skeletal muscle as the inactive b form. Thus, only the muscle enzyme is responsive to allosteric regulation via ATP and AMP, with high levels of AMP (signalling exercise) activating phosphorylase b and vice versa for ATP. Similarly, glucose works in the liver only to allosterically inactivate phosphorylase a due to the need to be responsive to blood glucose levels, rather than energy requirements.

8.4.2.3 Hormonal regulation by glucagon and adrenaline

Muscular contraction and sympathetic stimulation during exercise leads to the release of adrenaline. This acts in the skeletal muscles to increase glycogen breakdown, freeing up glucose for energy provision. This operates through adrenoreceptors in the membrane of cells, signalling to a subsequent second messenger cascade which:
- Phosphorylates the phosphorylase to its a form, making it ACTIVE.
- Phosphorylates the synthase to its b form, making it INACTIVE.

In the liver, glucagon is a much more important hormonal messenger. Instead of indicating need for energy, glucagon acts as a signal of fasting allowing the release of glucose into the circulation. The second messenger cascade is effectively the same.

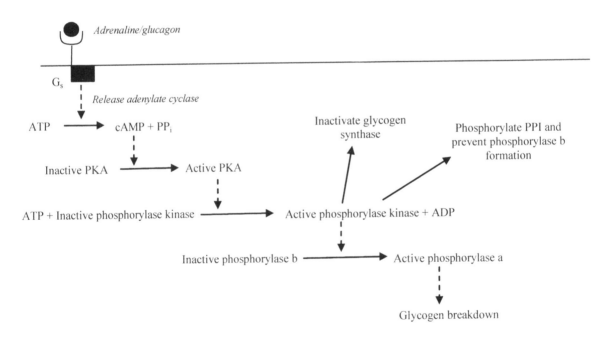

Figure 8.8 – Adrenaline/glucagon signalling cascade

8.4.2.4 Hormonal regulation by insulin

In a similar manner to glucagon and adrenaline, insulin acts on muscle and liver cells to increase the synthesis of glycogen. This occurs during high glucose levels and involves a tyrosine kinase-dependent second messenger cascade.

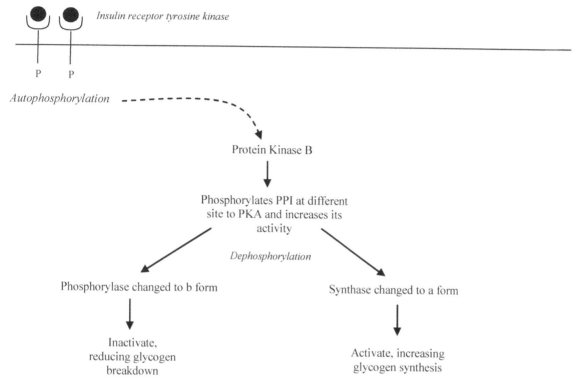

Figure 8.9 – Insulin signalling cascade

8.4.2.5 Regulation through calmodulin

In addition to the mechanisms described above, calcium regulation also plays an essential role in glycogen metabolism. This is particularly important in the skeletal muscle, where contraction is accompanied by a transient increase in intracellular calcium concentration:

1. Muscle contraction or electrical activity leads to release of calcium from endoplasmic or sarcoplasmic reticulum stores.
2. Calcium binds δ-calmodulin subunit of phosphorylase kinase.
3. Activation of phosphorylase kinase (moreso when enzyme phosphorylated – i.e. under influence of adrenaline and glucagon).
4. Activation of glycogen phosphorylase.
5. Breakdown of glycogen and release of glucose for energy provision in contracting muscles.

8.5 GLUCONEOGENESIS

Gluconeogenesis is the production of glucose from non-carbohydrate precursors, including lactate, pyruvate, TCA cycle intermediates, amino acids and glycerol. This occurs mainly in the liver and renal cortex, with these tissues being the only ones to possess glucose-6-phosphatase, and therefore able to release glucose from its glucose-6-phosphate derivative.

Under normal circumstances, the liver is a net producer of glucose, whilst other tissues are net consumers. Gluconeogenesis is particularly important for the brain and red blood cells (amongst others) as these rely on glucose as their major energy source.

8.5.1 Quantitative importance of gluconeogenesis
The daily requirements of glucose by various tissues are:

Tissue	Requirement
Brain	110g
Muscle	30g
Renal medulla	30g
Red blood cells	25g
Total	>195g

The average daily intake of glucose is only 100g, whilst liver glycogen (90g) and blood glucose (15g) only provide sufficient stores for around 12 hours of fasting. Therefore, glucose is too valuable a resource to be used unnecessarily. In order to reduce utilisation, and provide glucose during fast, other, more abundant dietary substrates must be used to synthesise glucose and maintain glycogen stores.

8.5.2 Substrates for gluconeogenesis
Gluconeogenesis can occur from a range of gluconeogenic substances, the main ones being lactate, alanine, glutamine and glycerol:
- Lactate – comes from anaerobic glycolysis in the muscle, renal medulla and red blood cells. This requires the Cori cycle to enter the liver.
- Alanine – under less extreme fasting conditions, the conversion of pyruvate to alanine by transamination is used to re-oxidise NADH in mitochondrial shuttles. In addition, a large amount may be released from muscle during a prolonged fast.
- Glutamine – during fasting, glutamine is produced from the muscle, catabolism of branched-chain polypeptides, other amino acids and glucose. This enters gluconeogenesis through α-ketoglutarate in the TCA cycle.
- Glycerol – glycerol is released from the hydrolysis of triglycerides, and enters gluconeogenesis by being converted to glyceraldehyde-3-phosphate (glycolytic intermediate).
- Other sugars – isomerisation or direct conversion to intermediates of the glycolytic pathway (e.g. fructose-1,6-bisphosphate from fructose).

In addition to glycerol, fatty acids are also released in triglyceride metabolism. These can not be used in gluconeogenesis since the conversion of pyruvate to acetyl CoA (a potential route of entry) is irreversible. Furthermore, going via the TCA cycle is impossible since two carbons are lost as CO_2, and thus the addition of carbons in the form of 2C acetyl CoA (from fatty acid break down) produces no net increase in the number of carbon molecules circulating. Thus, there is effectively no substrate from which glucose may be synthesised.

8.5.3 The gluconeogenic pathway
Gluconeogenesis from most substrates passes via pyruvate. Thus, it appears that gluconeogenesis is simply the reverse of glycolysis. However, due to irreversible steps in glycolysis catalysed by

84

hexokinase, phosphofructokinase and pyruvate kinase it is not. Instead, gluconeogenesis is described as a reciprocal pathway, with various reactions used to bypass those that are irreversible. This is essential since it prevents futile cycling.

Each of the enzyme-catalysed reactions of gluconeogenesis consume two molecules of ATP. Thus, the synthesis of a single glucose molecule requires 6 ATP, plus 2 NADH molecules. Considering glycolysis is only able to generate two ATP molecules directly, this highlights the need to input a large amount of energy in the short term to obtain ATP in the long term through aerobic respiration and the electron transport chain.

The pathway is as follows:

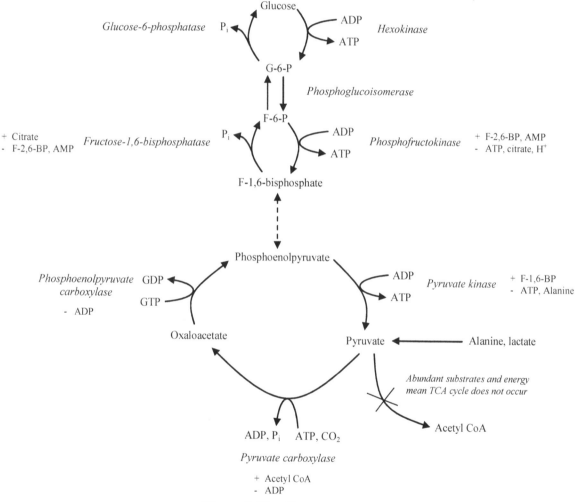

Figure 8.10 - Gluconeogenesis

8.5.4 Allosteric regulation of glycolysis and gluconeogenesis
Overall, glycolysis is regulated to occur when energy and substrate levels are low. Gluconeogenesis on the other hand occurs when energy and substrate levels are high, allowing synthesis of glucose and subsequent storage as glycogen. Obviously, the exception to this is low glucose levels, which stimulates gluconeogenesis and inhibits glycolysis.

Each of the enzyme-regulated steps of glycolysis and gluconeogenesis are reciprocally regulated – inhibition of one enzyme by an allosteric factor occurs concomitantly with the activation of the opposite enzyme with the same allosteric factor. As such, the irreversible steps of glycolysis (i.e. those whose release of free energy is such that the reverse reaction is kinetically impossible) are bypassed by alternative enzyme-regulated reactions in gluconeogenesis, and regulated to prevent futile cycling.

Reaction	Glycolysis enzyme	Regulation	Gluconeogenesis enzyme	Regulation
Glucose $\leftrightarrow$ G-6-P	Hexokinase	N/A	Glucose-6-phoshatase	N/A
F-6-P $\leftrightarrow$ F-1,6-BP	Phosphofructokinase	+ F-2,6-BP, AMP − ATP, citrate, H^+	Fructose-1,6-bisphosphatase	+ Citrate − F-2,6-BP, AMP
PEP $\rightarrow$ Pyruvate	Pyruvate kinase	+ F-1,6-BP − ATP, alanine	N/A	N/A
Pyruvate $\rightarrow$ Oxaloacetate	N/A	N/A	Pyruvate carboxylase	+ Acetyl CoA − ADP
Oxaloacetate $\rightarrow$ PEP	N/A	N/A	PEP carboxylase	− ADP

8.5.5 Hormonal regulation of glycolysis and gluconeogenesis
In addition to the above allosteric regulators, insulin, glucagon and cortisol are responsible for regulation on both an acute and chronic timescale.

Acute hormonal control involves glucagon and insulin. These hormones are released in response to circulating blood glucose levels, with a view to either increasing or decreasing glucose respectively.
- Glucagon – released in response to low glucose levels, and therefore increases gluconeo-genesis and decreases glycolysis. Glucagon acts via cAMP and PKA to phosphorylate and inactivate fructose-6-P:2-kinase (and therefore reduce the levels of fructose-2,6-bisphosphate) and pyruvate kinase (reducing the conversion of PEP to pyruvate)
- Insulin – released in response to high glucose, and therefore a hormone that should work to increase the rate of glycolysis. Insulin activates the synthesis of fructose-2,6-bisphos-phate, leading to strong stimulation of phosphofructokinase and strong inhibition of fructose-1,6-bisphosphatase. This is essential in preventing futile cycle (good example of reciprocal control) and ensuring solely glucose breakdown.

In response to prevailing conditions of high or low glucose, glucagon, insulin and cortisol can act to suppress or induce the transcription of the enzymes involved in glycolysis and gluconeogenesis. Again, the reciprocal activity of these enzymes ensures futile cycles are prevented over a more chronic timescale.

86

Hormone	Increase expression	Decrease expression
Insulin (promote uptake, use and storage of glucose)	Glycogen synthase Hexokinase Phosphofructokinase Pyruvate kinase	Pyruvate carboxylase PEP carboxylase F-1,6-bisphosphatase G-6-phosphatase
Glucagon and cortisol (synthesis of as much glucose as possible)	Pyruvate carboxylase PEP carboxylase F-1,6-bisphosphatase G-6-phosphatase	Glucokinase Pyruvate kinase

8.6 FUTILE CYCLES

Futile cycling describes when two metabolic pathways run simultaneously in opposite directions with no overall effect other than wasting energy. If glycolysis and gluconeogenesis were to be active at the same time, glucose would be converted to pyruvate by glycolysis and then converted back to glucose by gluconeogenesis. The only outcome of this would be an overall consumption of ATP. Thus, reciprocal regulation of irreversible reactions is essential to prevent this happening.

Futile cycles have a role in metabolic regulation, with reciprocal regulation allowing an oscillation between two substrates to be highly sensitive to an allosteric molecule through amplification of the signal. In addition, futile cycles do generate heat, and may be used to maintain temperature such as in bumble bees and hibernating animals.

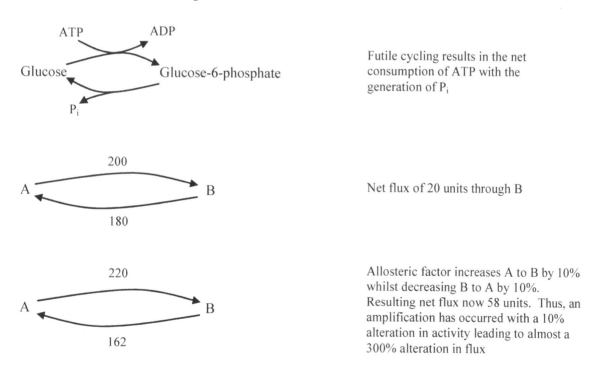

Futile cycling results in the net consumption of ATP with the generation of P_i

Net flux of 20 units through B

Allosteric factor increases A to B by 10% whilst decreasing B to A by 10%. Resulting net flux now 58 units. Thus, an amplification has occurred with a 10% alteration in activity leading to almost a 300% alteration in flux

CHAPTER 9

Amino Acid Metabolism

9.1 PROTEIN DIGESTION

The daily intake of protein from the diet is around 70-100g. In addition to the ingested proteins, 30-200g of protein in the form of digestive enzymes and shed intestinal epithelial cells are absorbed.

During digestion, proteins are broken down by peptidases:
- Endopeptidases – cleave bonds in the middle of the polypeptide.
- Exopeptidases – cleave either N-terminal (aminopeptidases) or C-terminal (carboxypeptidases) amino acids.
- Specific digestive enzymes including pepsin, trypsin and chymotrypsin.

Digestion of protein yields single amino acids, di-peptides and tri-peptides. These are taken up into intestinal epithelial cells and converted to free amino acids inside the cell (via peroxisomes and lysosomes) and released into the circulation.

Protein digestion in the stomach
There are two important components to the digestion of protein in the stomach:

1. Acid – H^+ ions secreted by parietal cells using the K^+/H^+-ATPase exchanger. This results in a lumen pH as low as 1. H^+ ions are produced from carbonic acid (formed by H_2O and CO_2 via carbonic anhydrase) whilst the potassium gradient is present due to diffusion out into the lumen.

2. Pepsins – these are proteolytic enzymes active at pH 2. Pepsins are secreted as pepsinogen precursors, which self-activate when the pH is below 5. Peptide fragments generated from the precursor cleavage are able to stimulate the duodenal wall to produce CCK – a hormone signal which induces pancreatic juice secretion.

Protein digestion by the pancreas
The pancreas secretes a 'juice' containing various proteolytic enzymes (active at neutral pH) and HCO_3^- which neutralises gastric acid.

The enzymes secreted include trypsin and chymotrypsin. Enterokinase from intestinal cells activates trypsinogen to trypsin, which is subsequently able to cleave additional trypsinogen. Chymotrypsinogen and precursors to elastase and carboxypeptidase A and B are also activated by trypsin.

9.2 AMINO ACIDS
Essential and non-essential
Amino acids may be classified as being either essential or non-essential. Essential amino acids are those which must be obtained in sufficient quantities from the diet. These are leucine, isoleucine, valine, phenylalanine, threonine, tryptophan, methionine, lysine and histidine.

The dietary intake of arginine is too low, and therefore this essential amino acid must be synthesised endogenously from other more abundant amino acids.

If any of the essential amino acids is omitted from the diet, then a negative nitrogen balance arises – nitrogen excreted being greater and nitrogen absorbed. This reflects the constant turnover of protein and obligatory amino acid metabolism if protein synthesis is impaired. The absence of one essential amino acid means that proteins containing that amino acid cannot be fully synthesised. As such, the entire incomplete polypeptide chain is excreted, resulting in a negative nitrogen balance which extends beyond merely a lack of one type of amino acid.

Fates of amino acids
Broadly, the fates of amino acids fall into four categories:
- Body protein synthesis – only amino acid store in the body.
- Oxidation for energy, such as in intestinal cells (glutamate used as a major energy source).
- Synthesis of hormones, neurotransmitters and pigments.
- Conversion to glucose or fatty acids for storage as glycogen or triglyceride (when ingestion exceeds requirement).

Categories of amino acid
Apart from body protein (which is relatively inaccessible), there are no stores for amino acids. Thus, amino acids are constantly degraded, with the removal of amino groups to yield a carbon skeleton. These carbon skeletons are then converted to one of six intermediates:
- Pyruvate
- Acetyl CoA
- α-ketoglutarate
- Succinyl CoA
- Fumarate
- Oxaloacetate

Those amino acids whose carbon skeleton may be converted to pyruvate, α-ketoglutarate, succinyl CoA, fumarate or oxaloacetate are termed gluconeogenic, since they may be used to synthesise glucose.

Those amino acids whose carbon skeleton feeds into acetyl CoA are termed ketogenic, being used for fatty acid synthesis.

9.3 Amino Acid Metabolism

9.3.1 Oxidation
In order that the carbon skeletons of amino acids may be used for generation of metabolic intermediates, their α-amino group must first be removed. This process is known as transamination. Subsequently, the glutamate generated by this reaction must be deaminated itself, generating α-ketoglutarate and ammonia (which must then be excreted). Thus, the oxidation of amino acids occurs in two stages.

9.3.1.1 Transamination
Transamination describes the process whereby the α-amino group from an amino acid is transferred to α-ketoglutarate, resulting in the generation of glutamate and the corresponding α-keto acid. These reactions are catalysed by transaminases, which are found predominantly in the liver – e.g. aspartate transaminase, alanine transaminase. Clinically, this is important since levels of these enzymes in the blood act as indicators of liver cell damage.

The oxidative deamination of glutamate uses NAD^+ as a coenzyme, with its reduction to NADH. Glutamate dehydrogenase is regulated allosterically, with GTP and ATP acting as inhibitors, whilst ADP and GDP act as activators. Thus, when energy levels in the cell are low (i.e. ADP and GDP are high), oxidative deamination occurs at a rapid rate, resulting in increased generation of α-ketoglutarate which may feed into the TCA cycle for energy generation.

9.3.1.3 Fate of ammonia generated
Since there is no store for nitrogen in the body, and ammonia is toxic, humans convert the ammonia generated in the deamination of glutamate to urea. This is a considerably more water soluble compound, and may therefore be freely excreted in the urine.

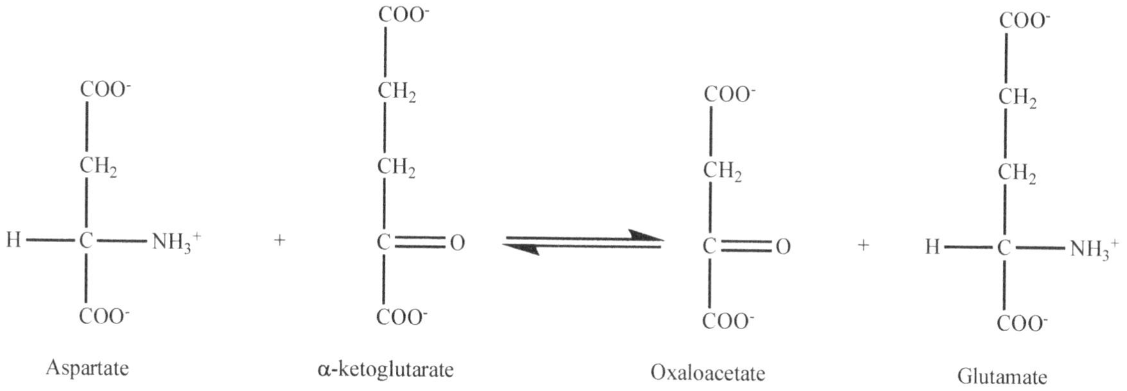

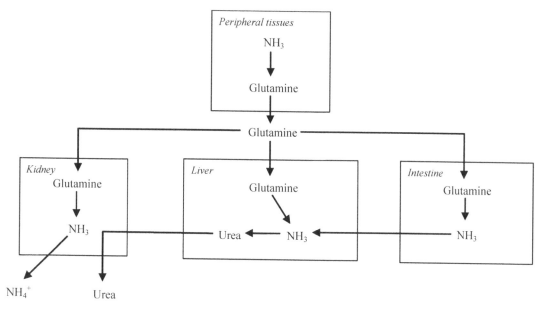

Figure 9.1 – Transamination of aspartate

Ammonia is important for normal animal acid-base balance. After formation of ammonium from glutamine, α-ketoglutarate may be degraded to produce two molecules of bicarbonate which may be used as buffers for dietary acids. In addition, ammonium is excreted in the urine resulting in net acid loss. Ammonia may itself diffuse across the renal tubules, combine with protons, and thus allow for further acid excretion by increasing the diffusion gradient.

9.3.1.4 Ammonia and glutamine in the peripheral tissues

Peripheral tissues are unable to generate urea themselves. Therefore, ammonia generated from the oxidation of amino acids must be transferred to the liver and converted to non-toxic urea (urea cycle – see below). Since the vast majority of amino acid metabolism takes place in the liver this only accounts for a small proportion of the total urea generated. Given the toxicity of ammonia to the brain, excess generated in peripheral tissues is converted first to glutamine, which is then transported to the liver (for urea synthesis), intestine and renal cortex (for energy generation).

Figure 9.3 – Nitrogen metabolism

In the renal cortex and intestine, glutamine may be used as a major energy source:

- Renal cortex – NH_3 generated from the conversion of glutamine to glutamate and subsequently α-ketoglutarate is excreted directly as NH_4^+ in the urine, playing a role in the acid buffering system.
- Intestine – glutamine is used as a major energy source, with the carbon skeleton being oxidised to CO_2 and H_2O. The NH_3 generated when glutamine is converted to glutamate and subsequently α-ketoglutarate, is released into the portal venous system as alanine and NH_4^+. This portal venous drainage delivers these compounds to the liver for the generation of urea.

9.3.2 Urea Synthesis

Since there is no store for nitrogen compounds in the body, nitrogen must be converted to ammonia (which is highly toxic) and then excreted as ammonia itself, uric acid or urea (in most terrestrial vertebrates). In order for this to occur, urea is synthesised by the liver via the urea cycle, and is then transported to the kidneys for excretion in the urine.

Overall, the reaction is:

$$NH_4^+ + HCO_3^- + H_2O + \text{Aspartate} \rightarrow \text{Urea} + \text{Fumarate}$$

(Uses 3ATP, with the generation of 2ADP, AMP, $2P_i$ and PP_i)

The detailed urea cycle is shown below. The initial step, generating carbomyl phosphate is rate limiting, and therefore central to regulation:

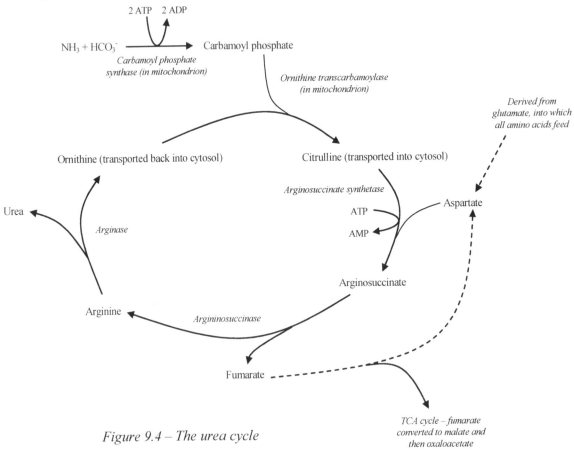

Figure 9.4 – The urea cycle

Site of urea synthesis
The urea cycle occurs mainly in the periportal cells of the liver lobules. The periportal cells are the outer part of the lobule, where NH_3 is converted to urea and where alanine, other amino acids and NH_3 may be taken up. The cells on the inner part of the lobule are near the portal venous system, and therefore are specialised for high rates of transamination, synthesising α-ketoglutarate and glutamine from glutamate.

Control of the urea cycle
Acute

- Acute control is exercised by alteration of enzyme activity.
- The controlled step of the urea cycle is the generation of carbomyl phosphate by carbomyl phosphate synthase.
- A specific activator of this enzyme, N-acetylglutamate is used for control.
- NAG is synthesised from glutamate and acetyl CoA by NAG synthase.
- Glutamate is used as a signal of nitrogen content of the cell, whilst acetyl CoA is a signal of energy charge.
- When lots of nitrogen needs to be excreted, and there is abundant energy, both glutamate and acetyl CoA are increased, leading to increased NAG and thus accelerated urea synthesis.

Chronic

- High protein intake induces an increase in synthesis of urea cycle enzymes, with a 3-4 fold increase in production over 24-36 hours.

9.3.3 Tissue-specific amino acid metabolism
Liver
The liver is the most important organ for amino acid metabolism, generating urea from ammonia and metabolic intermediates from the carbon skeleton.

After a meal, amino acid uptake is proportional to concentration (except for leucine, isoleucine, valine and citrulline). Between meals, 50% of hepatic uptake and 10-15% of glucose output is due to alanine.

Intestine
After meals, all amino acids from dietary proteins are taken up from the lumen. Virtually all the amino acids are subsequently released into the portal circulation (to be transported to the liver) in proportion to their concentrations. However, neither glutamine nor aspartate are released, since these are used for energy generation.

Between meals, glutamine is taken up from the peripheral circulation for energy. In addition, the gut synthesises alanine and citrulline from other amino acids and metabolic intermediates, releasing them into the peripheral circulation. Arginine in particular is released by the intestine, which is used by the liver for protein synthesis, urea formation and creatinine synthesis.

Kidney
The kidney takes up citrulline from the gut and synthesises arginine. Thus, in combination with the gut the urea cycle occurs. The kidney possess argininosuccinate synthase and argininosuccinase, whilst the gut contains carbomyl phosphate synthase, ornithine transcarbamoylase and arginase (compare with urea cycle diagram). The liver is the only organ in the body where the urea cycle occurs as a whole.

In addition, the kidney takes up glutamine, using it for energy, NH_3 generation and glucose synthesis.

Muscle

Muscle fibres use amino acids for energy, either directly or via pyruvate. Muscle exports alanine, glutamine and pyruvate to the liver for gluconeogenesis.

In addition, muscle selectively retains branched chain amino acids to prevent muscle wasting during fasting. Branched chain amino acids (especially leucine) are anabolic, increasing protein synthesis, insulin secretion and lactate release, whilst inhibiting muscle breakdown. This minimises damage during a glucose fast.

CHAPTER 10

Cellular Organisation of Metabolism

10.1 CELLULAR ORGANISATION OF METABOLISM

10.1.1 Overview
Eukaryotic cells contain a number of organelles, each of which contains a specialised environment in order to perform certain metabolic roles. Transport of molecules between these organelles allows integration of metabolism and functioning of the cell as a coherent unit:

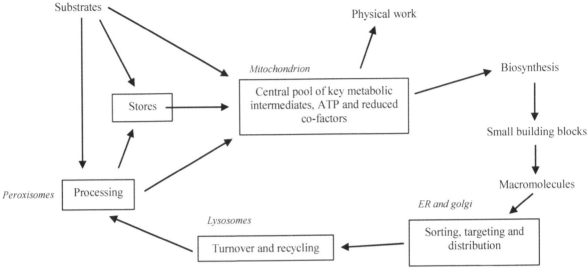

Figure 10.1 – Cellular organisation of metabolism

Compartmentalisation has its advantages and disadvantages:

Advantages

Clustering of related functions and compounds serving a common purpose, or requiring a common environment.

Isolation ensures controlled access and thus regulation (where transport controlled step).

Removal of potential harmful process and substrates from the general cell environment.

Disadvantages

Isolation requires transport mechanisms for substrates, products and intrinsic components of the compartment.

10.1.2 Mitochondria
Roles of mitochondria
Clustering of major energy forming reactions
- β-oxidation of fatty acids
- Pyruvate oxidation
- Oxidation of amino acids
- Urea formation in the liver

Generation of key metabolic intermediates and reduced cofactors
- Acetyl CoA
- TCA cycle intermediates
- NADH and FADH$_2$

Final common pathway of energy production
- Electron transport chain
- ATP synthase
- ATP and ADP translocation

Mitochondrial isolation – substrates and products
The outer membrane of mitochondria has transmembrane channels based on porin proteins. These make the membrane freely permeable to molecules with a molecular weight up to 10,000.

The inner membrane is highly selectively permeable, with no mechanism of carrying NADH, acetyl CoA or fatty acyl CoA – thus requiring shuttle systems
- Specific carriers are present for pyruvate, amino acids, ADP/ATP, inorganic phosphate, citrate, malate and α-ketoglutarate.
- Specific shuttle systems for NADH (aspartate shuttle), acetyl CoA and fatty acyl CoA (carnitine shuttle).

Mitochondrial isolation – genetic and proteins
Mitochondrial proteins are almost all synthesised from nuclear genes. Thus, they are produced in the cytoplasm and must be taken up into the organelle (requiring specific N-terminal leader sequences). The uptake of mitochondrial proteins also requires inner membrane receptors and energy in the form of a proton gradient.

Once imported, the N-terminal leader sequences are cleaved from the protein and folding and assembly may take place using chaperonins.

Mitochondrial genome and disease
The mitochondrial genome consists of 16,500bp in circular DNA. It is maternally transmitted and there are approximately 10,000 copies per cell. The genome codes for 13 subunits of electron transport chain components, 22 tRNAs and some rRNAs. In conjunction with nuclear proteins, the genome is able to undergo replication, transcription and mRNA processing and gene product translation. The arrangement and functioning of the genome provides evidence for mitochondria representing symbionts – subcellular organisms that inhabited eukaryotic cells at some point in their evolution.

There are various (maternally transmitted) mitochondrial diseases, including MELAS and MERRF. These result in myopathies (characterised by proximal muscle weakness, eyelid drooping and cardiac problems) with death finally occurring from cardiac arrhythmia. Histologically, mitochondrial disease results in the accumulation of ragged red muscle fibres, due to the overproduction of mitochondria to compensate for their ineffective function, and the subsequent accumulation of these mitochondria at the cell membrane.

10.1.3 Endoplasmic Reticulum/Golgi Apparatus
The ER and Golgi apparatus form a continuous secretory vesicle system.

Roles of the ER and Golgi
Biosynthesis
- Synthesis of phospholipids, glycolipids, membranes, complex carbohydrates and glyco-proteins – particularly important for membrane component synthesis.

Targeting and distribution
- Glycosylation signals on proteins for distribution to cell membranes, lysosomes and extracellular export.

Detoxification
- Contain the cytochrome P450 hydroxylating system.
- Family of enzymes which all catalyse monooxygenase reactions – insertion of an oxygen atom into a substrate, with the other oxygen generating water.
- Electrons used to generate water are passed down a series of transporters linked to P450 enzymes, which use NADPH as the ultimate electron donor.

Protein import into the ER is done using leader sequence recognition, as with mitochondria. Docking of ribosomes with the ER allows the translation of proteins directly into the organelle (rough ER).

10.1.4 Lysosomes
Roles of lysosomes
Lysosomes play a particularly important role in degradation and recycling:
- Re-use of macromolecule monomers
- Degradation of foreign particles, such as bacteria
- Re-use of DNA/RNA, proteins, complex sugars and lipids

Lysosomal enzymes
The operation of lysosomes is based upon a large set of acid hydrolases, including nucleases, proteases, lipases and glycosidases:
- All work at optimal pH ~4.8, which is generated by the lysosome proton pump.
- Acid environment favours the denaturation of macromolecules for degradation.
- Products released into the cytoplasm.

Targeting and disease
Proteins destined for the lysosome are synthesised by the RER, with the addition of mannose residues. Mannose-6-phosphate within these targeted proteins is recognised by the Golgi such that they are enclosed within clathrin-coated vesicles. These vesicles are transported towards lysosomes, with which they fuse, allowing enzyme and acid access to the macromolecule.

This mechanism of delivery is important also for the degradation and processing of extracellular substances, such as cholesterol in LDL or bacterial antigens. A failure of lysosomal enzymes can lead to a build up of macromolecules, leading to diseases in which brain damage, skeletal and facial deformities occur.

10.1.5 Peroxisomes
Roles of peroxisomes
Processing by oxidation (e.g. of very long chain fatty acids and D-amino acids)
- Oxidation does not generate ATP as in mitochondria, but instead forms toxic H_2O_2.
- As such, oxidation is coupled with the action of enzymes such as catalase, superoxide dismutase and glutathione peroxidase contained within the peroxisome, which catabolise H_2O_2 to water and oxygen.

Biosynthesis
- Plasmalogens for cells membrane and bile acids (e.g. cholic acid) from cholesterol.

Gluconeogenesis
- Conversion of otherwise unusable compounds into gluconeogenic precursors e.g. D-amino acids into α-keto acids.

Zellweger Syndrome
Almost everything that is known about peroxisomes comes from study of this disease, in which peroxisomes are non-functioning. Zellweger syndrome has a neonatal onset, and death occurs within months. Babies are born floppy, unresponsive and demonstrate repeated seizures.

The disease is characterised by cortical defects (due to the presence of unnecessary structures leading to deformation), jaundice, fibrosis, cholestasis, siderosis, renal cysts and adrenal hypoplasia.

10.2 BIOCHEMICAL PRINCIPLES OF NUTRITION

10.2.1 Macronutrients
There are four broad components to nutrition:
- Micronutrients (<1g/day) – vitamins and minerals
- Macronutrients (>1g/day) – carbohydrates, fats, protein and fibre
- Water
- Oxygen

Typically, the daily macronutrient intake consists of:
- Carbohydrates (~300g/day) – polysaccharides, disaccharides and monosaccharides
- Fats (~100g/day) – triacylglycerols, phospholipids and cholesterol
- Proteins (~100g/day)
- Fibre (~10-20g/day)

10.2.1.1 Dietary carbohydrate
The different types of dietary carbohydrate are measured by glycaemic response (change in plasma blood glucose over time, after ingestion of a certain type of food). This is particularly important for diabetics since it enables them to predict their blood glucose levels.

Starch (e.g. white bread)
- Consists of amylose and amylopectin.
- Amylose can crystallise, such as in potatoes, making it harder to digest.
- Has low glycaemic response, with small but sustained increase in blood glucose levels (important for diabetics).

Glucose and other monosaccharides
- Very high glycaemic response, with prolonged excess leading to type II diabetes.

Fibre
- Non-starch polysaccharide.
- Has no glycaemic response since it is able to pass through the digestive system without being absorbed.
- Plays a similar role to 'resistant starch' which is also not absorbed.

Fermentation of some carbohydrates by gut bacteria can lead to the production of short chain fatty acids, such as acetate and proprionate, which may subsequently be absorbed.

10.2.1.2 Dietary fatty acids
Broadly there are three different types of fatty acid, each of which has their own nutritional benefit.

Saturated fats e.g. palmitic acid
- Have the effect of raising serum cholesterol.
- Tend to be associated with insulin resistance since saturated fats make membranes less fluid, and therefore impair detection mechanisms.
- Increase the likelihood of developing coronary heart disease and other vascular conditions.

Monounsaturated fats e.g. oleic acid
- Lower serum cholesterol.
- Increase the relative amounts of HDL and are thus beneficial in preventing vascular disease.

Polyunsaturated fats e.g. linoleic acid
- Essential in diet as can not be synthesised endogenously.
- Lower serum cholesterol, but also lower HDL cholesterol levels.
- Overall, decrease the likelihood of developing CHD.
- n-3 PUFA – typically found in vegetable oils. Lower cholesterol and are pro-inflammatory.
- n-6 PUFA – typically found in fish oils. Lower serum triacylglycerol, reduce platelet aggregation, stabilise heart rhythm and are anti-inflammatory. Protective against heart disease and other vascular conditions.

10.2.2 Micronutrients
10.2.2.1 Vitamins
A vitamin is an organic compound required in tiny amounts for essential metabolic reactions in a living organism. Most vitamins cannot be obtained in sufficient quantities by endogenous synthesis, and therefore must be obtained from the diet. Vitamin deficiency results in characteristic diseases.

Vitamin	Biochemical role	Effect of deficiency/disease
Niacin (vitamin B_3)	Precursor to NAD^+ and $NADP^+$ – metabolism and DNA repair	Pellagra
Riboflavin (vitamin B_2)	Precursor to FAD and FMN – metabolism of fats, carbohydrates and proteins	Growth retardation
Pyridoxine (vitamin B_6)	Production of monoamine neurotransmitters (serotonin, dopamine, adrenaline and noradrenaline)	Anaemia
Thiamine (vitamin B_1)	Precursor to thiamine pyrophosphate – important in carbohydrate and fat metabolism	Beriberi
Folic acid (vitamin B_9)	Precursor to tetrahydrofolate – required for DNA synthesis	Megaloblastic anaemia Neural tube defects
Vitamin B_{12}	Precursor to deoxyadenosyl cobalamin – required for DNA synthesis, myelin sheath formation and fatty acid metabolism	Megaloblastic anaemia

10.2.2.2 Minerals

Iron
See chapter 11.

Zinc
Dietary intake
- Zinc is found in oysters, and to a far lesser degree in most animal proteins, beans, nuts, almonds, whole grains, pumpkin seeds and sunflower seeds.
- The recommended dietary allowance of zinc post-puberty is 11mg for males and 8mg for females. Higher amounts are recommended during pregnancy and lactation.

Distribution
- It is estimated that up to 3,000 proteins in the human body contain zinc prosthetic groups, of which the zinc finger is the most common.
- Over a dozen types of cells in the human body secrete zinc ions, and zinc ions are now considered neurotransmitters.
- Cells of the salivary glands, prostate, immune system and intestine are particularly notable examples.

Biological roles
- Zinc prosthetic groups e.g. zinc finger
- Neurotransmitter
- Secretion from certain cells
- Activator of some enzymes e.g. carbonic anhydrase
- Deficiency can result in hair loss, skin lesions, diarrhoea and tissue wasting. Deficiency in utero impairs brain development.

Copper
Dietary intake
- Rich sources of copper include oysters, beef or lamb liver, brazil nuts, cocoa, and black pepper.
- The RDA for normal healthy adults is 0.9mg/day

Distribution and biological roles
- Copper is carried mostly in the bloodstream on a plasma protein called ceruloplasmin.
- When copper is first absorbed in the gut it is transported to the liver bound to albumin.
- Copper is found in a variety of enzymes, including the prosthetic centres of cytochrome c oxidase and superoxide dismutase.
- In addition to its enzymatic roles, copper is used for electron transport.
- Copper facilitates iron uptake, and therefore deficiency disease is characterised by anaemia-like symptoms.

10.3 CLINICAL BIOCHEMICAL MEASUREMENT
Types of measurement
Various parameters may be measured from a multitude of bodily fluids and compartments (e.g. blood, saliva, CSF, semen, expired gas etc.)
- Gases e.g. O_2, CO_2 – diagnosis of respiratory failure
- Ions e.g. Na^+, K^+, Cl^-, Ca^{2+}
- pH – diagnosis of diabetic ketoacidosis etc.

- Osmolality – dehydration or fluid overload
- Metabolic substrates e.g. high glucose, ketones – diagnosis of diabetes
- Hormones e.g. diabetes, Cushing's syndrome
- Enzymes – isoenzymes and tissue damage, metabolic diseases etc.

Enzyme measurement
Enzyme measurement can be used to assess tissue damage and enzyme deficiencies, amongst other conditions:
- Cardiac and liver enzymes for diagnosis of MI, cirrhosis, hepatitis etc. – lactate dehydrogenase, pyruvate kinase, creatine kinase, aspartate transaminase etc.
- Enzyme deficiencies – high levels, but ineffective or insufficient production.

Enzymes may be used in the laboratory to assess the level of biologically-important molecules. For example, glucose assays employ glucose oxidase or hexokinase, whose rate of reaction is proportional to sample glucose levels. These two enzymes produce by-products in these reactions which may be measured and correlated with patient blood glucose levels.

CHAPTER 11

The Liver in Metabolism

11.1 OVERVIEW

In metabolism, the liver is involved in:

- Glucose homeostasis – storage of glycogen as an energy reserve and the conversion of other metabolic intermediates to glucose via gluconeogenic reactions.
- Fat metabolism – β-oxidation in the liver, synthesis of triglycerides from excess sugars and amino acids and the production of ketone bodies from fatty acids for their use in other tissues as an energy source.
- Amino acid metabolism – oxidation of amino acids via transamination reactions and the synthesis of body proteins, glucose and fatty acids from amino acids.
- Urea synthesis – urea cycle in the periportal cells of the liver lobule allowing the conversion of ammonia from peripheral tissues into urea and other compounds.

Other functions of the liver include plasma protein synthesis, trace element homeostasis, detoxification, alcohol metabolism, vitamin and cofactor metabolism and storage (e.g. of iron containing compounds).

11.2 HEPATIC PROTEIN SYNTHESIS: EXAMPLES

11.2.1 Albumin

Albumin is a plasma protein with a heart-shaped structure containing three homologous domains. It has a concentration of 4500-5000mg/dL in the blood.

Capillary walls are relatively impermeable to albumin and other plasma proteins, meaning that these plasma proteins are able to exert an osmotic force of 25mmHg across the capillary wall. This is known as the oncotic (colloid) pressure. The oncotic pressure operates in capillary beds to pull water back in from interstitial compartments, and thus regulate the fluid balance between intravascular and tissue spaces:

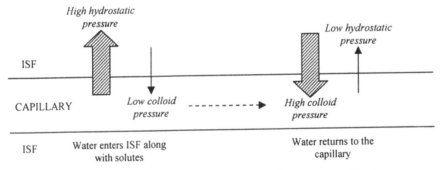

Figure 11.1 – Osmotic and oncotic forces in capillaries

Oedema

Oedema is the abnormal accumulation of large amounts of interstitial fluid. If the pressure in the capillaries exceeds the oncotic return, then there is a net flow of fluid out of the capillary leading to fluid accumulation.

There are a number of causes of oedema:

1. Increased hydrostatic pressure due to arteriolar dilation, venular constriction, heart failure increasing venous pressure and gravity (e.g. during long-haul flights).

104

2. Decreased oncotic gradient across the capillary due to decreased plasma protein levels. This can occur in liver failure, Kwashiorkor or decreased dietary protein. Also, the accumulation of osmotically active substances in the interstitial spaces (e.g. Na^+ and Cl^- in congestive cardiac disease) can have the same effect.
3. Increased capillary permeability via substance P, histamine, kinins and other substances.
4. Inadequate lymphatic flow leading to lymphoedema. This may be caused by removal of lymph nodes (e.g. axillary node retrieval in breast cancer surgery) or blockage, such as through parasitic worms. Parasitic lymphoedema often presents as massive swelling of legs and scrotum, and may be treated with drugs that increase macrophage proteolysis of albumin.

Albumin and transport
Albumin functions as a transporter for thyroid, adrenocortical, gonadal and other hormones. Binding to these hormones prevents them from being rapidly filtered through glomeruli in the kidney, and represents a stable reservoir of hormones that can be accessed.

Albumin also serves as a transport for metal ions, shorter chain fatty acids, amino acids, bilirubin, enzymes and some drugs. Other liver-synthesised transport proteins include transferrin, used in the mobilisation of iron around the body.

11.2.2 Vitamin K-dependent Clotting Factors
Vitamin K-dependent clotting factors (II, VII, IX and X) are all protease enzymes that work in the clotting cascade to sequentially activate each other, resulting in the generation of an insoluble fibrin polymer from fibrinogen.

The synthesis of these clotting factors in the liver occurs with the help of vitamin K. Vitamin K acts as a co-factor for the enzyme that converts glutamic acid residues into γ-carboxyglutamate, giving the factors their metal ion binding function. Inhibition of this process by medication such as warfarin is used in the treatment of hypercoagulable states and anti-thrombotic prophylaxis.

In liver disease, clotting factor synthesis may be deranged. Obstructive jaundice leads to a lack of bile in the intestine. This subsequently depresses fatty acid absorption, and thus the absorption of fat-soluble vitamin K (amongst other vitamins). Thus clotting factors V, VII, IX and X are not synthesised properly. Furthermore, cirrhotic disease of the liver prevents the proper synthesis of these clotting factors.

The liver is also involved in the synthesis of a variety of proteins which inhibit the effect of vitamin K-dependent clotting factors and other zymogens in the clotting cascade:
- α-1-antitrypsin – protease inhibitor.
- Antithrombin III (combined with heparin), which binds to and blocks serine proteases.
- Protein C and protein S which inactivate factors V and VIII, whilst increasing plasmin formation.
- Plasmin from inactive plasminogen precursor (converted through the action of thrombin and tissue plasminogen activator - t-PA)

11.3 IRON TRANSPORT AND STORAGE

11.3.1 Absorption
The average daily intake of iron is around 20mg. However, the amount absorbed is only equal to

losses, representing 3-6% of the total amount ingested. Absorption occurs mainly in the upper part of the small intestine, particularly the mucosal cells of the duodenum and jejunum.

In its ferrous (Fe^{2+}) state, iron is readily absorbed. However, most dietary iron is in the ferric (Fe^{3+}) form. Very little iron is absorbed in the stomach therefore, but gastric contents aid in the dissolution of iron and its conversion to the ferrous form through ascorbic acid complex formation. This has been demonstrated with the high frequency of iron deficiency anaemia in patients post-gastrectomy surgery.

Absorption of iron also occurs as haem. The ferrous iron that haem contains is released in the mucosal cells of the gastrointestinal tract. Haem is highly soluble, and therefore absorption is much more efficient and rapid than non-haem iron.

Absorption of non-haem iron occurs in multiple steps within the GI tract:
1. Iron binds to mucin of the mucous overlying enterocytes.
2. Brush border integrin transfers the iron to mobilferrin molecules, which carry the iron into cells. The number of available sites on mobilferrin determines the amount taken up into the cell. Thus, iron deficiency leads to an increase in available sites (and thus iron uptake capacity) whilst overload has the opposite effect.
3. Enterocytes contain iron-binding apoferritin which supplies mitochondria with iron.
4. The iron not absorbed into mitochondria remains bound to apoferritin (forming ferritin) or the iron is transferred to the protein transferrin in the plasma.

11.3.2 Transport and Distribution
Apoferritin (storage)
- Apoferritin combines with iron with the cell to form ferritin.
- Iron bound to ferritin is lost when cells are shed into the gastrointestinal lumen.
- Ferritin molecules exist as micelles of ferric hydroxyphosphate, which can contain up to 4500 Fe atoms.
- Ferritin acts as the principle store of iron through the body, with ferritin molecules within lysosomal membranes able to aggregate and form deposits known as haemosiderin (representing a large iron store). Ferritin is also found in the plasma.
- Ferritin represents around 25% of body iron.

Transferrin (transport)
- Transferrin is the iron-transporting polypeptide within the plasma.
- Transferrin has two iron binding sites, and is normally ~35% saturated within the plasma, at a concentration of 23μmol/L.
- The amount of transferrin in the plasma is inversely proportional to the amount of iron in the body. Thus, low iron levels stimulate an increase in transferrin to increase the transportation capacity of the plasma.
- The greater the transferrin saturation (and thus, the greater the total body iron), the more iron that enters mucosal cells to be bound to ferritin and lost via cell shedding.

11.3.3 Homeostasis of Iron
In adults, the amount of iron lost from the body is very small and these losses are generally unregulated. Total body iron stores merely change according to variations in the rate of iron absorption by the intestine. On average, men lose around 0.6mg per day, whilst in women losses vary with menstruation.

Dietary factors may alter the absorption of iron:
- Ratio of haem to non-haem iron.

- Phytic acid found in cereals, phosphates and oxalates react with iron to make it non-absorbable.
- Pancreatic juice inhibits iron absorption such that fatty meals, which stimulate exocrine pancreatic activity, can prevent absorption.

Loss of iron occurs through:
- Shedding of gastrointestinal cells.
- Bleeding.

11.3.4 Consequences of Excess and Deficiency

High iron	Low iron
- Mobilferrin binds to less iron	- Mobilferrin binds to more iron
- Decrease in circulating transferrin and increased transferrin saturation	- Increase in circulating transferrin and decreased transferrin saturation
- Increased storage within cells as ferritin and thus increased loss through cell shedding	- More iron moved to plasma, being released from ferritin stores thus reducing losses from mucosae
- Decreased rate of iron absorption	- Increased absorption when stores are depleted (or erythropoiesis taking place)
- Extreme excess → haemosiderosis followed by haemochromatosis with skin pigmentation and various organs becoming affected	- Extreme deficiency → anaemia

11.4 DETOXIFICATION

Detoxification reactions involve the conversion of toxic, lipophilic compounds into polar, more water soluble derivatives for excretion. Modifications include the introduction of functional groups through oxidation and reduction, and conjugation to new functional groups.

11.4.1 Oxidation/Reduction Reactions

Oxidation and reduction reactions are important in the detoxification of compounds in liver microsomes.

Dehydrogenase reactions
- Dehydrogenases (such as alcohol dehydrogenase) use NAD^+ to oxidise compounds. In the case of alcohol, ethanol is converted to the carboxylic acid derivative in tight coupling with aldehyde dehydrogenase:

$R\text{-}CH_2\text{-}OH + NAD^+ \rightarrow R\text{-}CHO + NAHD/H^+$ Catalysed by alcohol dehydrogenase

$R\text{-}CHO + NAD^+ + H_2O \rightarrow R\text{-}COOH + NADH/H^+$ Catalysed by aldehyde dehydrogenase

- The second of these reactions generates a carboxylic acid which may be excreted in the urine.

Reductase reactions
- Reductase enzymes use NADPH as a cofactor to react with aldehydes, ketones, quinines, azo-, nitro- and nitroso- compounds.

Oxidase reactions
- Oxidase enzymes use FAD as a cofactor.
- Since these reactions generate H_2O_2 as a by-product, they occur in the peroxisomes such that the hydrogen peroxide may be broken down.
- Substances detoxified in this manner include amines:

$$R\text{-}CH_2\text{-}NH_2 + O_2 + H^+ + H_2O \rightarrow R\text{-}CHO + NH_4^+ + H_2O_2 \qquad H_2O_2 \text{ broken down by catalase}$$

11.4.2 Mono-oxygenase Reactions

Mono-oxygenases comprise the endoplasmic reticular cytochrome P_{450} system. The P_{450} system represents a small electron transport chain, with the aim of modifying toxic compounds. This consists of a complex series of flavoproteins and cytochromes, each using NADPH as an electron donor and molecular oxygen with the resultant hydroxylation of compounds.

This system of reactions can operate on almost every compound, and thus serves an important role in drug metabolism:
- Alkanes and alkenes e.g. aflatoxin
- Aromatic hydrocarbons e.g. naphthalene
- Heterocyclic amines e.g. quinolone
- Amides e.g. urethane
- Ethers e.g. indomethacin
- Sulphides e.g. chlorpromazine

Mono-oxidases containing flavin are highly non-specific and contain flavoproteins, but no cytochromes. These enzymes are used for the detoxification of amines such as propranolol, morphine and nicotine.

Unfortunately, not all the reactions catalysed by the cytochrome P_{450} system lead to detoxification. Some result in the activation of xenobiotics (foreign substances) to more toxic compounds. This is particularly relevant for carcinogens, which may only become active after passing through this system of enzymes. However, the same activating reactions are used to convert inactive forms of a drug (e.g. those which may be ingested) into derivatives with therapeutic activity.

The cytochrome P_{450} system may be induced by particular substances, thus interfering with the metabolism of other unrelated compounds. For example, the metabolic inactivation of oral contraceptive hormones occurs in women also taking rifampicin or barbiturates.

11.4.3 Conjugation

Conjugation involves the incorporation of functional groups by oxidation/reduction reactions. These functional groups provide receptor sites for the conjugation of additional groups, and increase the solubility and reactivity of the target compound. Commonly used groups in conjugation include:
- Glucuronic acid
- Sulphate
- Acetyl groups
- Amino acids

Glucuronidation
- Glucuronic acid consists of a glucose molecule with a COOH group instead of an aldehyde moiety. UDP is used to activate it before reaction with compounds.
- May act on endogenous compounds (e.g. bilirubin, steroid hormone metabolites) and exogenous substances (e.g. chloramphenicol, morphine).

Sulphation
- Addition of sulphate groups uses PAPS (3-phospho-AMP-sulphate) as a functional group donor.

Amino acids
- In the addition of amino acids (normally glycine) the target molecule is first activated with CoASH.
- Benzoic acid (used as a preservative) is detoxified in this manner.

11.5 ALCOHOL METABOLISM

Cirrhosis of the liver is the 6th to 9th commonest cause of disease in the Western world, with alcohol being the causative agent in 41-95% of cases. The liver is particularly susceptible to alcohol since it is the primary site of metabolism, and thus sacrifices itself to preserve function in other organs. Most of the toxic effects of alcohol are due to acetaldehyde and NADH, with metabolic effects including hypoglycaemia, lactic acidosis and hyperuricaemia.

11.5.1 Hepatic Alcohol Metabolism

Metabolism of alcohol in the liver involves a single oxidation of CH_3CH_2OH to CH_3CHO. This is reaction is catalysed by alcohol dehydrogenase (cytosol), the P_{450} system (ER) and catalase (peroxisomes)

Cytoplasmic alcohol dehydrogenase
- This is the most important process in alcohol metabolism.
- The enzyme consists of around 20 isoenzymes, derived from over 7 genes, allowing for variable expression and activity of different isoenzymes. This may account for variations in susceptibility to alcohol.
- The reaction catalysed by alcohol dehydrogenase uses NAD^+:

$$CH_3\text{-}CH_2\text{-}OH + NAD^+ \rightarrow CH_3\text{-}CHO + NADH/H^+$$

Cytochrome P_{450} – 2E1 mono-oxygenase
- This enzyme is induced by alcohol ingestion, and is located particularly in the centrilobular hepatocytes of the liver.
- The location of this enzyme leads to the pattern of liver damage where central cells of the lobule get most damaged in cirrhosis.
- Induction by alcohol means there may also be increased conversion of xenobiotics to toxic compounds, leading to increased susceptibility to solvents.
- In chronic alcohol ingestion, this pathway of detoxification predominates over ADH.
- The reaction using the mono-oxygenase uses $NADPH/H^+$:

$$CH_3\text{-}CH_2\text{-}OH + NADPH/H^+ + O_2 \rightarrow CH_3\text{-}CHO + NADP^+ + 2H_2O$$

Catalase
- Peroxisomal catalase plays a minor role in ethanol metabolism:

$$CH_3\text{-}CH_2\text{-}OH + H_2O_2 \rightarrow CH_3\text{-}CHO + 2H_2O$$

11.5.2 Acetaldehyde Dehydrogenase

Having generated $CH_3\text{-}CHO$ from alcohol metabolism, the liver needs to dispose of this intermediate.

Over 90% of acetaldehyde metabolism is performed by acetaldehyde dehydrogenase, but the normal biological role of this enzyme is probably to metabolism aldehyde intermediates from biogenic amines.

Acetaldehyde dehydrogenase has four main classes, with I and III present in the cytoplasm, and II and IV in the mitochondria. The main enzyme in alcohol metabolism is mitochondrial II, and therefore acetaldehyde must be transported from the cytoplasm to mitochondria.

Variations in the four types of enzymes can be held responsible for different reactions to alcohol. 50% of Chinese and Japanese people experience flushing, hypotension and tachycardia on alcohol ingestion due to a type II variant that is less active. This reaction may lead to an aversion to alcohol, but continual drinking regardless leads to liver damage due to acetaldehyde accumulation.

11.5.3 The Toxic Effects of Alcohol
The toxic effects of alcohol are due mainly to acetaldehyde, acetate and NADH. In addition, alcohol may modify the metabolism of certain drugs.

Acetaldehyde
- Causes mitochondrial dysfunction, lipid peroxidation, increased collagen synthesis (causing scarring and fibrosis).
- Leads to synthesis of neo-antigens, to which the immune system responds.
- Decreases microtubule function leading to altered transport and secretion.
- Effects of acetaldehyde are due to the formation of protein adducts as it is able to react spontaneously with amino groups of lysine residues in proteins.

Acetate
- Acetate is the end product of alcohol metabolism after acetaldehyde breakdown.
- Breakdown reaction causes a significant increase in AMP levels which, when converted to uric acid, may crystallise leading to gut motility problems and gout.
- Must be treated with allopurinol.

NADH
- Decreases fatty acid oxidation, leading to fat storage and thus fatty liver.
- Increases triglyceride synthesis, leading to a fatty liver.
- Increases cholesterol synthesis via the proliferation of the ER.
- Inhibits gluconeogenesis, leading to depletion of glycogen stores and hypoglycaemia.
- Increases lactate levels, leading to lactic acidosis.
- Decreases albumin secretion through a microtubule effect.
- Increases hepatocyte size.
- Increases collagen synthesis, leading to liver fibrosis.

Drug metabolism modification
- Induction of the cytochrome P_{450} system increases the metabolism, and thus decreases the half-life of drugs including warfarin, phenytoin, phenobarbital and propranolol.
- Increases activation and toxicity of paracetamol, isoniazid, cocaine, carbon tetrachloride and various carcinogens.

11.6 CATABOLISM OF HAEM
Haem is part of a group of compounds known as tetrapyrole pigments. It is present in the prosthetic group of both α and β-globin and in the cytochromes of the electron transport chain. The functional part of the haem group is an Fe^{2+} ion, which can form co-ordinate bonds or undergo redox reactions.

11.6.1 Pathway of Degradation

The pathway of degradation of red blood cells leads to the release of haem, which must then undergo reactions to enable it to be excreted:

1. Ageing red blood cells lyse, releasing their haemoglobin into the plasma, via the tissue macrophage system.

2. Globin portion of haemoglobin is split off, leading to the release of haem.

3. Haem oxygenase in the spleen and liver carries out oxidative ring opening of haem, to produce the green substance biliverdin. Haem oxygenase is a cytochrome P_{450} enzyme, and uses NADPH and O_2. The iron released is recycled for haemoglobin synthesis.

4. Biliverdin reductase converts biliverdin to bilirubin.

5. Bilirubin binds to albumin in the plasma to allow it to be transported around the body. Some of it is tightly bound, but most dissociates allowing free bilirubin to enter liver cells and bind to cytoplasmic proteins. There is competition for the albumin binding sites with certain drugs.

6. Bilirubin is conjugated with glucuronic acid in hepatocytes using glucuronyl transferase, present in the smooth endoplasmic reticulum. This forms bilirubin diglucuronate with UDPGA, which is far more soluble than normal bilirubin.

7. The highly soluble conjugated bilirubin is actively transported into bile canaliculi for excretion in the bile. Since bilirubin is responsible for the colour of bile, obstruction to the biliary tree can lead to pale stool.

The intestinal mucosa is relatively impermeable to conjugated bilirubin, but is much more permeable to bilirubin itself and urobilinogens (a group of colourless compounds formed by the action of intestinal bacteria on bilirubin). This means that some of the bile pigments and urobilinogens are reabsorbed into the portal circulation, with some being excreted again by the liver, some entering the general circulation and some passing into the urine.

11.6.2 Jaundice

When bilirubin accumulates in the blood, the skin, sclera and mucous membranes turn yellow. This yellowing is known as jaundice and is detectable when the total plasma bilirubin is greater than $34\mu mol/L$. Hyperbilirubinaemia (and thus jaundice) may be caused by:
- Excess bilirubin production e.g. due to haemolytic anaemia.
- Decreased bilirubin uptake by hepatocytes.
- Disturbed intracellular protein binding or conjugation.
- Disturbed bilirubin secretion into bile canaliculi.
- Intra and extrahepatic bile duct obstruction.

The first three of these causes of jaundice lead to an elevation in free unconjugated bilirubin in the plasma. The last two lead to an increase in the levels of conjugated bilirubin. Thus, the causes of jaundice can be detected through liver function tests, which include the relative levels of conjugated and unconjugated bilirubin.

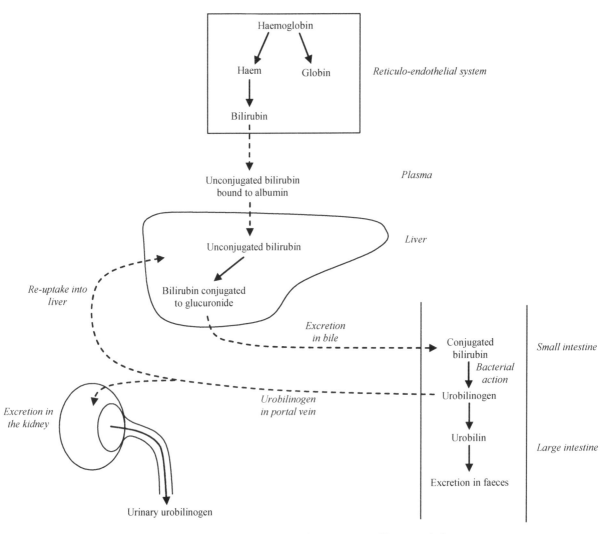

Figure 11.2 – Breakdown and excretion of haemoglobin

Kernicterus
Kernicterus is a neurological syndrome resulting from unconjugated bilirubin being deposited in the basal ganglia of the brain. This happens rarely in adults, but may happen in neonates due to:
- Increased blood-brain barrier permeability in infancy.
- Immature bilirubin conjugating system in infancy.

Kernicterus is a particular problem in children born with haemolytic diseases, such as erythroblastosis or haemolytic disease of the newborn.

11.7 LIVER FUNCTION TESTS
Liver function tests are often performed in the clinical setting in order to:
- Detect the presence of liver disease.
- Detect the type of liver disease such that more extensive investigation may be performed.
- Follow the progress of liver disease.

112

Test	Function
Bilirubin in blood and urine	Hepatic anion transport.
Plasma bilirubin fractions	Normally 95% of plasma bilirubin is unconjugated, but certain types of liver disease may lead to conjugated formed predominating.
Alanine aminotransferase (ALT) in blood	Soluble cytoplasmic enzymes are released in hepatocyte damage. However, both ALT and AST are located in periportal cells, so do not give a reliable indication of central damage. Also, there is a 24 hour lag-time.
Aspartate aminotransferase (AST) in blood	Both cytoplasmic and mitochondrial isoenzymes, so released more than ALT in chronic liver disease.
Alkaline phosphatase (ALP) and γ-glutamyl transferase (GGT)	Anchored in hepatocyte membrane, so not released in cellular damage. Much greater release when there is cholestasis (e.g. in gallstones) since there is a higher enzyme synthesis due to the presence of bile acids.
Hepatic protein synthesis	Albumin – decrease is a sign of chronic liver disease, but care must be taken since the half life of albumin is 20 days and there are other causes of decreased levels e.g. nutrition. Prothrombin time – deficiency in prothrombin and clotting factor synthesis causes an increased prothrombin time. This occurs in all liver disease since the half life is only 6 hours. This may also be caused by vitamin K deficiency.

11.8 THE CONSEQUENCES OF LIVER FAILURE

Liver failure may be caused by a number of processes, including alcoholic cirrhosis and chronic infection. There are significant and life-threatening effects of liver failure:

1. Hypoglycaemia due to impaired gluconeogenesis and glycogen breakdown.
2. Decrease in plasma urea since the liver fails to convert excess amino acids to urea. This occurs late in liver disease.
3. Raised concentrations of plasma lipid fractions if cholestasis is present.
4. Jaundice and associated toxic effects.
5. Decreased triglyceride levels as less is being created from excess sugars and amino acids. Also, decreased ketone body synthesis so some other organs suffer.
6. Decreased amino acid oxidation, leading to their accumulation.
7. Lowered plasma albumin leading to oedema and ascites (fluid in the abdominal cavity).
8. Increased sensitivity to drugs, alcohol and other toxins since the liver is unable to perform detoxification reactions.
9. Reduced storage of iron ferritin compounds, leading to anaemia if dietary intake of iron is not sufficient or absorption is impaired.

CHAPTER 12

Lipoproteins

12.1 FATS AND LIPIDS

Lipids are essential as structural components of membranes, as a major energy source and as precursors for steroid hormones, prostaglandins and leukotrienes. Fatty acids may be synthesised by the liver, or derive from dietary intake. Their storage in adipose tissue is in the form of glycerol esters (triglyceride), such that in the fasting state they may be released for energy production.

There are many human diseases which can affect the absorption or distribution of lipids in some way, leading to symptoms due to disturbance in the above functions.

Fat is used as a metabolic fuel preferentially in certain tissues for a number of reasons:
-   Large stores (75% of total energy stores).
-   Can be completely depleted without compromising body function.
-   Rapid metabolism and turnover.
-   Ideal for tissue with high, sustained energy requirements such as the heart, renal cortex and liver.
-   Highly concentrated as hydrophilic clumps in stores, unlike glycogen which is 60% water.
-   Energy per gram content is high since fat is reduced.

However, the metabolism of fat also carries a number of disadvantages:
-   Insoluble in water, meaning it requires special adaptations for use and transport in aqueous environments.
-   Can not be converted to glucose which is problematic for red blood cells, the renal medulla and eye since these are anaerobic areas, and thus require glucose for metabolism.
-   Can not be metabolised by the brain, although ketone bodies may be produced though these are rarely sufficient.

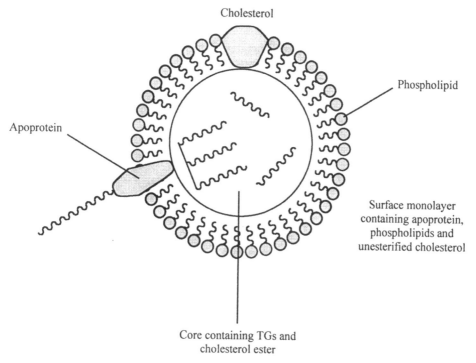

Figure 12.1 – Lipoprotein structure

12.2 Lipoproteins

Free fatty acids may be transported bound to albumin in the plasma. However, triglycerides are too hydrophobic to be transported in this manner, so have to be packaged with cholesterol and apoproteins by hepatocytes and enterocytes. This forms structures known as lipoproteins, with a central core containing triglycerides and cholesterol esters, and a surface monolayer coat containing apoprotein, phospholipids and unesterified cholesterol. The surface layer makes the lipoprotein water soluble.

Lipoproteins are released into the plasma, where they undergo stepwise enzymatic degradation in order to release triglycerides into the tissues. When within the plasma, they can change their components, size and shape as well as their constituent apoproteins. Alteration in apoprotein allows certain cells around the body to take up certain apolipoproteins via cellular receptors.

There are five broad classes of lipoprotein, increasing in density from chylomicrons to high density lipoprotein. The density of the particles is inversely proportional to the triglyceride content, but proportional to the protein content.

Particle	Source/function	Main Component	Apoprotein	Mechanism of Lipid Delivery
Chylomicron	Made in intestine Transports dietary lipid	Triglyceride (99%)	B48 (strains A, C and E)	Lipoprotein lipase hydrolysis
Very low density lipoprotein (VLDL)	Made in liver Transports endogenous synthesised lipids	Triglyceride	B100 (A, C and E)	Lipoprotein lipase hydrolysis
Intermediate density lipoprotein (IDL)	Derived from VLDL	Triglyceride and cholesterol	B100 (E only)	Internalised by liver and converted to LDL
Low density lipoprotein (LDL)	Derived from VLDL and IDL Transport of cholesterol	Cholesterol	B100	Internalised by liver and other tissues via LDL receptors
High density lipoprotein (HDL)	Made in liver Reverse cholesterol transport	Proteins	AI and AII (C and E)	Transfer of cholesterol esters to IDL and LDL

12.2.1 The Exogenous Lipid Cycle

Lipoprotein metabolism consists of the exogenous and endogenous cycles, each of which is centred on the liver. The cycles are interconnected and involve two key enzymes:
- Lipoprotein lipase – releases free fatty acids and glycerol from chylomicrons and VLDL into the tissues.
- Lecithin cholesterol acyl transferase (LCAT) – forms cholesterol esters from free cholesterol and fatty acids.

116

12.2.1.1 Assimilation and Transport of Dietary Fatty Acids
The major problem of lipid digestion for animals is their insolubility in water. To overcome this, dietary fat is assimilated in three stages:

1. Emulsification – lipolytic enzymes of pancreatic juice are water soluble, so can only act on the outside of a lipid droplet. Thus bile salts are used to emulsify the lipid droplets, since bile contains detergent substances such as cholic acid, to increase the surface area exposed to enzyme.

2. Digestion – most digestion occurs in the duodenum and small intestine with pancreatic lipase (a Ca^{2+}-requiring enzyme) breaking down the 1 and 1' fatty acids from a triglyceride, producing two fatty acids and one monoglyceride. Less than 10% of the original triglycerides remains unhydrolysed.

3. Absorption – due to their high lipid solubility, fatty acids, monoglycerides and diglycerides are able to readily diffuse across the brush border of microvilli in a process that is not protein mediated. Once inside epithelial cells, the products of digestion move to the smooth ER aided by fatty acid binding protein (FABP).

12.2.1.2 Reprocessing in the sER – Formation of Chylomicrons
Within the sER, monoglycerides re-esterify with fatty acids to form triglyceride molecules:
- Requires conversion of fatty acids to fatty acyl CoA in a reaction catalysed by fatty acyl CoA synthetases.
- Requires energy for bond formation which is provided by the cleavage of the thioester bond of fatty acyl CoA.
- Triglycerides are formed by the transfer of the fatty acyl group from CoA derivatives to the glycerol backbone in a reaction catalysed by fatty acyl CoA transferase.

The reprocessed lipids, together with phospholipids and proteins are packaged into large lipoprotein chylomicrons consisting of:
- 88% triglyceride
- 8% phospholipid (though 80% of outer shell)
- 3% cholesterol ester
- 1% cholesterol
- 1-3% apoproteins A, B48, CII and E

12.2.1.3 Transport of Chylomicrons
Chylomicrons are exocytosed by the cell and enter the lateral spaces between the cells. Being too large to pass through the basement membrane of the capillaries around the mucosa, chylomicrons enter the lymphatic system (lacteals) since their fenestrations are large enough for uptake.

Chylomicrons leave the intestine in the lymph, mainly entering the thoracic duct. They pass into the venous circulation and thereby bypass the liver and arrive at peripheral tissues directly.

12.2.1.4 Release of Fatty Acids from Chylomicrons
Triglycerides are unable to pass directly into the interstitial fluid from capillaries, and therefore must be hydrolysed by lipoprotein lipase (LPL) to monoglycerides and fatty acids to be absorbed.
- LPL is found on the outer surface of endothelial cells of capillaries in some tissues.
- Presence demonstrated by the ability of heparin to bind to the component of endothelial

cells which holds LPL in place, with the subsequent release of the enzyme into the circulation. Heparin is itself a large anionic structure that can bind to LPL.

Having been released by LPL, fatty acids are taken up by cells of peripheral tissues for use in hydrolysis or are recombined with triglycerides for storage in adipose tissue. Glycerol is transported to the liver for further metabolism.

The breakdown of the chylomicron by LPL leads to the depletion of triglyceride content, whilst the outer surface substances are lost to HDL. The chylomicron remnant is taken up by the liver, which recognises ApoE and forms vesicles which fuse with lysosomes. The remnants are degraded into constituent amino acids, fatty acids and free cholesterol. The lipids that are delivered to the liver are then synthesised into VLDLs and returned to the plasma.

Medium and short chain fatty acids of less than 10 carbons are released into the portal blood and bind to albumin. Albumin has 10 binding sites for fatty acids, 3 of which are of high affinity. Bound to albumin, the fatty acids are transferred to the liver. This accounts for over 99% of free fatty acid. Triglycerides containing medium chain fatty acids are useful in patients with malabsorption problems as they can be absorbed in tact and hydrolysed completely without being re-esterified by entereocytes.

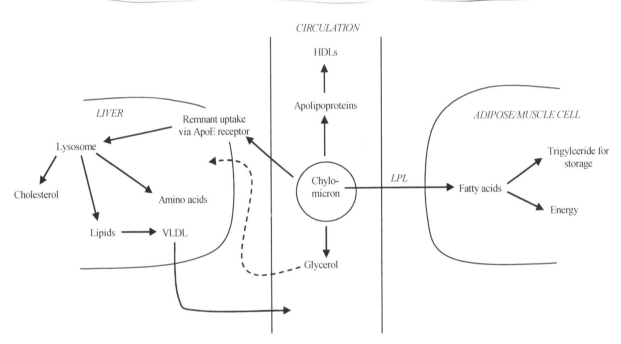

Figure 12.2 – Chylomicron breakdown

12.2.2 The Endogenous Lipid Cycle

The endogenous lipid cycle describes the movement of fatty acids and cholesterol, packaged in various different lipoproteins, between the liver, peripheral tissues and adipose stores:

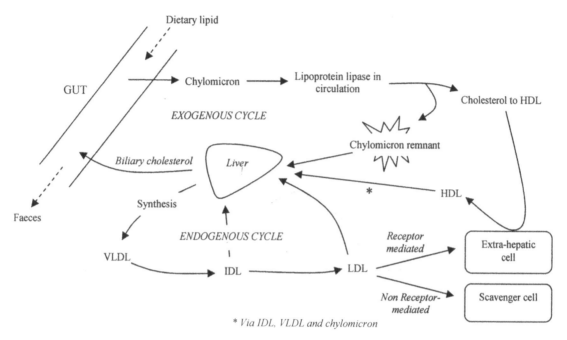

Figure 12.3 – The endogenous and exogenous lipid cycles

12.2.2.1 VLDL and IDL Metabolism

Metabolism of VLDL is the first stage in the endogenous lipid cycle. Endogenously synthesised triglycerides are transported by VLDL, which is synthesised in the liver on a backbone of ApoB100. During synthesis, the binding of triglycerides to the protein backbone is facilitated by microsomal triglyceride transfer protein (MTP). In the circulation, the cholesterol contained within VLDLs is transferred to HDL particles which esterify it in a process catalysed by LCAT (lecithin cholesterol acyl transferase). During synthesis of VLDLs within the liver, this esterified cholesterol is transferred back to VLDL (thus setting up a loop), using cholesterol ester transport protein (CETP), in exchange for triglycerides.

Once synthesised, VLDL particles enter the circulation. As with chylomicrons, VLDLs are broken down in the periphery by lipoprotein lipase, which hydrolyses the triglycerides to form a VLDL remnant. This remnant is smaller than VLDL and contains relatively more cholesterol and ApoE. At this stage, some of the VLDL is internalised back into the liver, of which some is converted to IDLs by hepatic triglyceride lipase.

The IDLs that are generated may be taken up by the liver or converted to LDL particles. 75% of the IDLs are taken up by the liver via receptors that recognise ApoE and ApoB100. The other 25% is converted to LDL by hepatic lipase, with the loss of all apoproteins except B100, which is essential in LDL binding.

119

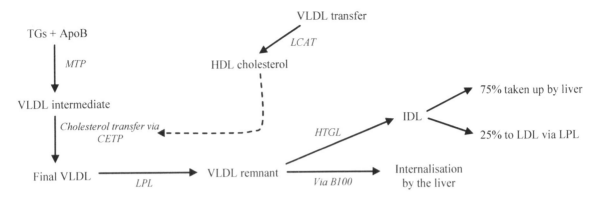

Figure 12.4 – VLDL metabolism

12.2.2.2 LDL Metabolism

LDL metabolism is the final step in VLDL metabolism. LDL consists of an oily core with 1500 cholesterol ester molecules and a hydrophilic shell of phospholipid, cholesterol and ApoB100. The primary function of LDL is to deliver cholesterol to extrahepatic tissues for cell membrane synthesis, steroid and vitamin D synthesis. Thus, tissues possess both a receptor-mediated and non-receptor-mediated LDL uptake pathway, with the latter being more important in high LDL scenarios. Receptor-mediated uptake, which occurs through the ApoB100 and ApoE proteins, involves endocytosis and is regulated in relation to the needs to the cell. Problems with the ApoB100 receptor lead to familial hypercholesterolaemia.

Receptor-mediated LDL uptake
- All nucleated cells contain the LDL (ApoB100) receptor.
- These receptors are located in regions of the cell known as 'coated pits' whose intracellular side is lined with clathirin – a protein that polymerises to stabilise the pit.
- Endocytosis of the LDL results in an endocellular vesicle coated in clathrin being formed. The clathrin coat is subsequently shed to form an endosome.
- The endosome is converted into a compartment with internal pH 5.0-5.5 which enables the LDL to dissociate from its receptor.
- Receptor-rich regions of the endosome bud off and return to the plasma membrane.
- LDL-containing endosomes fuse with the lysosome, allowing degradation of apoproteins to amino acids and cholesterol esters to free cholesterol and fatty acids.

Regulation of LDL receptors
- When the cell has sufficient cholesterol, LDL receptor synthesis is down-regulated.
- When insufficient cholesterol is available, receptors are upregulated.
- Absence or problem within the receptors can cause familial hypercholesterolaemia.
- Mutations in ApoB100 results in defective binding of LDL to its receptor and causes familial defective apoB (FDB).

Non-receptor-mediated LDL uptake
- The uptake of LDL by receptor-mediated mechanisms accounts for 75% of uptake, whilst the remaining 25% is taken up by low affinity scavenger receptors on macrophages.
- These receptors have a low affinity for LDL, but are specific to certain forms (particularly oxidised LDL).

- The synthesis of scavenger receptors is not regulated, so uptake of oxidised cholesterol occurs in an unregulated manner.
- As cholesterol in the cell accumulates, the macrophages form into foam cells. The build up of foam cells within blood vessel walls leads to the formation of fatty streaks which may develop into atherogenic plaques (potentially leading to heart attacks and strokes).

12.2.2.3 Cholesterol Removal from Cells

The VLDL-IDL-LDL cascade described above leads to the delivery of endogenously synthesised lipids to the peripheral tissues. The reverse process is mediated by HDL particles.

HDLs are synthesised from precursors, which are disc-shaped bilayers secreted by the gut and liver. HDLs are rich in surface components (i.e. phospholipids, apoproteins, cholesterol) but contain little core cholesterol ester or triglyceride. Two important forms of HDL exist – HDL 2 and HDL 3. HDL 2 is larger, with a higher cholesterol content whilst HDL 3 is smaller, with less cholesterol and a higher capacity for peripheral cholesterol than HDL 2. Interchange between these two occurs in the liver via hepatic lipase.

In addition to 'reverse' cholesterol and triglyceride transport, HDLs also serve as a repository for ApoC and ApoE which may be transferred between HDLs and to other lipoproteins as needed. ApoA is not exchanged since it is only present within HDLs.

HDLs acquire free cholesterol from peripheral tissues and transfer it to IDLs and chylomicron remnants, which are subsequently taken up by the liver such that the excess cholesterol may be excreted:
1. Uptake of cholesterol by HDL mediated by ApoA1 binding to cells.
2. Esterification of HDL cholesterol occurs, catalysed by LCAT.
3. Transfer of cholesterol esters to VLDL, IDL or chylomicron remnants by CETP.
4. Uptake of cholesterol-enriched particles by the liver, mediated by ApoE and B.

12.3 CLINICAL CONSIDERATIONS

Given the importance of regulation of lipid levels, it is unsurprising that derangements in any one of the processes outlined above can lead to clinical syndromes, each associated with particularly symptoms and effects.

12.3.1 Abnormalities in Lipid Digestion and Absorption

Failure to digest and absorb fats leads to excretion of excessive amounts, in the form of steatorrhoea (foul-smelling, non-solid, fatty stool, typically defined as being when fat excretion in faeces is in excess of 0.3 g/kg/day). This is most commonly caused by bile salt deficiency, such as in liver disease, or obstruction to the bile duct. In addition, it is seen in pancreatic enzyme deficiency (e.g. pancreatitis, cystic fibrosis) or defective chylomicron synthesis. Malabsorption of fats can lead to a deficiency in the fat soluble vitamins (A, D, E and K).

12.3.2 Hyperlipoproteinaemias

The normal range of plasma cholesterol concentrations vary amongst populations. However, there is a strong correlation between increased cardiovascular risk and increasing cholesterol levels. Hyperlipoproteinaemias are characterised by high cholesterol or triglyceride levels, and may be primary (i.e. genetic) or secondary.

Familial hypercholesterolaemia
- Inherited defect in the LDL receptor.
- 1 in 500 people are heterozygous for the FH gene.
- Carriers for FHC have cholesterol levels twice that of normal.
- Homozygotes have cholesterol levels 5-8 times that of normal.
- Large number of mutations have been found in the LDL receptor gene, which can result in problems with synthesis, transport to membrane, binding of LDL and clustering of receptors in clathrin pits.
- Affected individuals have premature cardiovascular disease, and stigmata of disease e.g. tendon xanthomata in the hands, xanthelasma around the eyes.

Type 1 hyperlipoproteinaemia
- Characterised by hypertriglyceridaemia.
- Caused by inability to clear chylomicrons from the plasma due to LPL and ApoCII deficiency.

Secondary causes of hyperlipoproteinaemia include hypothyroidism, diabetes mellitus, liver disease and alcohol abuse. These may be controlled by changes in lifestyle e.g. exercise and smoking cessation.

12.3.3 Lipid-lowering Medication
Various medical treatments are available for patients with hyperlipoproteinaemias, whether these be primary or secondary in cause.

HMG-CoA reductase inhibitors – 'Statins'
- Examples include simvastatin, pravastatin and atorvastatin.
- Analogues of HMG-CoA that inhibit the synthesis of cholesterol.
- HMG-CoA reductase catalyses the rate limiting step in cholesterol synthesis, and thus inhibiting the enzyme decreases hepatic cholesterol synthesis. This in turn decreases the synthesis of LDL receptors, and increases the clearance of LDL cholesterol from the plasma.

Bile resins
- Examples include cholestyramine and cholestipol.
- Sequester bile acids in the intestine, thus reducing absorption of exogenous cholesterol and increasing the metabolism of endogenous cholesterol to bile salts.

Pancreatic lipase inhibitors
- Examples include orlistat.
- Prevent the breakdown to lipids in the small intestine by lipases secreted by the exocrine pancreas.

12.3.4 Other Lipid-Based Diseases
In addition to those outlined above, there are many pathological processes and distinct diseases which rely on lipids in their development and thus their detrimental effects.

Disorder	Accumulated Lipid	Characteristic Features
Obesity	Triglyceride (adipose)	High risk of cardiovascular disease and diabetes
Atherosclerosis	Cholesterol (blood vessels)	High risk of cardiovascular disease and stroke
Fatty liver	Triglyceride (liver)	Commonly caused by chronic alcohol intake
Cholelithiasis	Gallstones (biliary tree)	Cause impaired lipid absorption
Ketoacidosis	Ketones (blood)	Occurs in uncontrolled diabetes, starvation and alcoholism
Carnitine deficiency	Triglyceride (many cells)	Impaired fatty acid oxidation
Sphingolipidosis	Partially degraded sphingolipids	Lysosomal hydrolase deficiency
Refsum's disease	Branched chain fatty acids (brain)	Peroxisomal enzyme deficiency

CHAPTER 13

Insulin and Diabetes Mellitus

13.1 INSULIN

Insulin is a small protein, consisting of two polypeptide chains (A and B chains) linked by two disulphide bonds. The A chain is 21 amino acids long, whilst the B chain is 30 amino acids long. Insulin has an essential role in the regulation of metabolism, integrating the usage of various substrates in different tissues around the body at different times.

13.1.1 Production of Insulin

Insulin is synthesised from a larger polypeptide called preproinsulin, which is cleaved soon after synthesis to form proinsulin. Proinsulin is then packaged into vesicles in β-cells of the islets of Langerhans and converted to insulin by cleavage of a connecting peptide (C-peptide), forming two distinct peptide chains. These peptide chains are released from cells by exocytosis in response to increases in glucose. Insulin is secreted directly into the hepatic portal vein, and thus reaches the liver directly since it has a short half-life of just a few minutes in the blood.

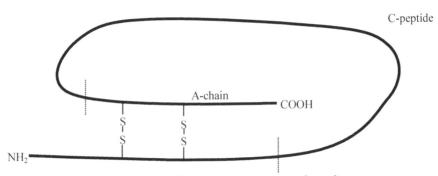

Figure 13.1 – Schematic structure of insulin

13.1.2 Secretion of Insulin

Insulin is secreted from β-cells in a mechanism dependent on calcium and potassium flow. Some medications used in the treatment of diabetes target this mechanism, facilitating or increasing insulin release:

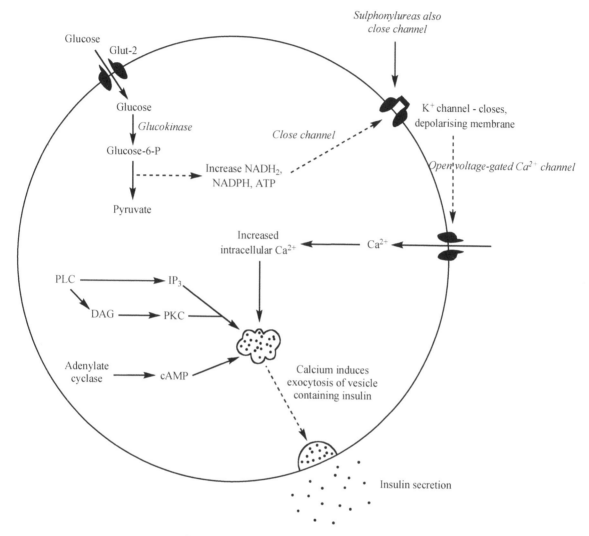

Figure 13.2 – The secretion of insulin

The release of insulin is stimulated by:
- High glucose in the blood
- Gastric inhibitory peptide
- Glucagon
- Sulphonylurea drugs (e.g. tolbutamide)
- Parasympathetic nervous activity

Insulin release is conversely inhibited by:
- Adrenaline

-   Somatostatin
-   Sympathetic autonomic activity

The release of insulin occurs rapidly initially, with pre-formed cell-contained hormone being release. There is then a longer phase of release of newly synthesised peptide.

13.1.3 Mode of Action
Insulin lowers blood glucose by facilitating uptake into muscle and adipose tissue, whilst simultaneously inhibiting hepatic glucose output.

The insulin receptor is a tetramer made of 2 α and 2 β glycoprotein subunits. α-subunits bind to insulin, whilst β-subunits span the membrane and have tyrosine kinase activity.
1.   Binding of insulin.
2.   Autophosphorylation of β-subunit tyrosine residues.
3.   Phosphorylation and dephosphorylation of certain cytoplasmic and membrane proteins, such as insulin-receptor substance 1 (IRS 1).
4.   Activation of Ras/Raf and subsequently MAP kinase cascades.
5.   Covalent modification of proteins, including transcription factors.
6.   Stimulation of synthesis of GLUT4 transporters and their migration and incorporation into the membrane. Also, stimulation of ion transport, amino acid uptake, lipid metabolism, effects on protein synthesis and degradation and glycogen synthesis and metabolism.

The activity of the above pathway is affected by overexposure to insulin (leading to desensitisation), the number of receptors (which increases in starvation) and adrenal hormones (excess glucocorticoids decrease receptor affinity).

13.1.4 Main Effects on Metabolism
The main effects of insulin on metabolism around the body are summarised in the table below:

Glucose/glycogen	Increase glucose entry
	Increase glycogen synthesis
	Decrease gluconeogenesis
	Increase glycolysis
Amino acids	Increase protein synthesis
	Decrease protein degradation
	Decrease release of gluconeogenic amino acids
	Increase transport of amino acids
Fatty acids	Increase fatty acid synthesis
	Increase triglyceride deposition
	Activate lipoprotein lipase
	Inhibit hormone-sensitive lipase
	Increase ketone uptake
	Increase lipid synthesis
Others	Increase uptake of K^+ into cells, lowering plasma K^+
	Increase cell growth
	Increase in mRNA for certain enzymes

126

13.2 DIABETES

Diabetes insipidus
- Diabetes insipidus is caused by a failure of vasopressin section or when the target organs (i.e. kidneys) do not respond.
- Can be due to neoplastic lesions in the hypothalamus or problems with the pituitary gland (cranial DI) or problems in the kidneys, such as congenital malfunction of V_2 receptors (nephrogenic DI).
- Leads to the production of vast amounts of watery urine (polyuria) and patients drinking large amounts of water (polydipsia).

Diabetes mellitus I
- Also known as juvenile onset diabetes mellitus.
- Patients have low plasma insulin and require injections.
- Probably due to autoimmune destruction of β-cells, triggered by childhood viral infection or due to amylin protein, that reduces insulin.
- Some toxins, drugs and surgery can lead to DMI.
- Caused by pancreatitis, haemochromatosis and Cushing's disease.
- Anti-islet cell antibodies (found in 90% of patients) react with β-cells and destroy them – this autoimmune mechanism explains why patients with certain human leukocyte antigens (HLAs) are more susceptible to developing the disease.

Diabetes mellitus II
- Generally presents in older patients (>40 years).
- Measurable levels of insulin present, but metabolic defect appears to lie either in defective insulin secretion or insulin resistance.
- Appears to be strong genetic link to the disorder, but there is little relationship to HLAs or immune mechanisms.
- May be due to a reduction in the insulin receptors in cells around the body in response to chronically high sugar or fat diet.

Secondary diabetes is the name given to diabetes caused by certain drugs, endocrine disorders and pancreatic problems (i.e. not those originating in autoimmune destruction of the pancreas). This includes the contraceptive pill, salbutamol and other catecholaminergic drugs, thiazide diuretics, Cushing's disease, acromegaly and pancreatitis.

	Type I diabetes	Type II diabetes
Prevalence	• 0.5% of population in Western World • Number of people affected is increasing	• 2-5% of population in Western World • Incidence increases markedly with age and varies with ethnicity
Typical age of onset	• *Juvenile onset*: between 1 and 25 years	• *Mature onset*: >40 years
Aetiology	• Irreversible autoimmune destruction of the pancreatic β-cells • Little or no insulin secretion	• Insulin is secreted, but in amounts that are inadequate to prevent hyperglycaemia or there is resistance to its action
Symptoms	• Polyuria, thirst and glucosuria • Marked weight loss and tiredness • Ketoacidosis	• Associated with obesity • Symptoms tend to be less acute than those in Type I diabetes

Genetics	• Polygenic • Concordance in monozygotic twins 40%. Associated with a mutation in a codon in the HLA DR3/4 gene causing autoimmune phenotype • β-cell destruction due to inflammatory reaction in islets triggered by environmental factors in genetically susceptible individuals e.g. viral infections (immune cross reactivity) and cow milk protein (molecular mimicry)	• Polygenic • Genetic component significant • Possible connection to calpain 10 – a protease, which may have some role in insulin secretion • Association with increased birth weight and early sensitivity of insulin receptors
Treatment	• Insulin	• Diet, exercise and lifestyle • Insulin releasing agents e.g. Sulphonylureas • Insulin sensitising agents e.g. metoformin • α-glucosidase inhibitors

13.2.1 Metabolic Disturbances in Uncontrolled Diabetes

13.2.1.1. Hyperglycaemia
Uncontrolled diabetes leading to hyperglycaemic attacks can cause symptoms due to hyperosmolarity of the blood. In addition, it results in glycosuria, with large amounts of glucose excretion in the urine coupled to a loss of water (osmotic diuresis) with polyuria. The resultant dehydration from the polyuria activates central signals, leading to increased water intake, known as polydipsia. In addition to loss of glucose in the urine, high urine output also leads to a loss of sodium and potassium which carries its own problems.

Other complications from hyperglycaemia include:
-   Glycosylation of small amounts of haemoglobin A to form HbA1c – this is used clinically as a marker of long-term diabetic control, comparing the effects and efficacy of insulin treatment.
-   Intracellular hyperglycaemia which activates the enzyme aldose reductase, increasing the synthesis of sorbitol and reducing cellular synthesis and activity of the Na^+/K^+-ATPase transporter.
-   Intracellular glucose can lead to the formation of advanced glycosylation end-products (AGEs) which are able to cross-link matrix proteins. Sorbitol and AGEs may play a role in the development of long-term microvascular and neurological problems in uncontrolled diabetes.

13.2.1.2 Protein Metabolism
In uncontrolled diabetes, the rate at which amino acids are catabolised to water and carbon dioxide increases. In addition, more amino acids are converted to glucose in the liver due to perceived starvation.
-   Dextrose to nitrogen ratio (D/N) gives an indication of the rate of gluconeogenesis from amino acids. For example, a ratio of around 3:1 in diabetes suggests 33% of the carbon from protein is being converted to glucose.

In uncontrolled diabetes, the increase in gluconeogenesis from protein is caused by:

128

- Glucagon increase leading to hyperglucagonaemia.
- Elevated adrenal glucocorticoids.
- Increased blood amino acid levels since no insulin is available to stimulate protein synthesis.
- Increased activity of the enzymes that convert pyruvate and other 2-carbon fragments into glucose (e.g. PEP carboxylase).
- Increased supply of acetyl CoA since there is no lipogenesis, which stimulates pyruvate carboxylase and the conversion of pyruvate to oxaloacetate.

The result of all the above is a net negative nitrogen balance, leading to protein depletion and muscle wasting. The combination of protein depletion and hyperglycaemia also makes diabetics more susceptible to infection, since some micro-organisms grow better in high glucose media.

13.2.1.3 Fatty Acid Metabolism
In uncontrolled diabetes, there is accelerated fat metabolism, increased ketone body formation and a decrease in fatty acid and triglyceride synthesis. Under normal conditions, 30-40% of ingested glucose is converted to fat, but in DM less than 5% is converted.

Complications and mechanisms of alterations in fat metabolism:
- Decreased conversion of glucose to fatty acids due to a decreased intracellular glucose concentration.
- Insulin inhibits hormone sensitive lipase in adipose tissue and thus, without insulin, the level of free fatty acids more than doubles.
- Increased glucagon leads to increased free fatty acids.
- Fatty acids are catabolised to acetyl CoA in the liver and other tissues. This outstretches the body's demand, whilst there is also an impairment in its conversion to malonyl CoA (a step required in fatty acid synthesis). This leads to an accumulation of acetyl CoA, which is converted to ketone bodies.
- Increased plasma concentration of triglycerides and chylomicrons due to decreased lipoprotein lipase activity, leading to lipaemic plasma.

13.2.1.4 Ketoacidosis
Due to the alterations in fatty acid metabolism outlined above, excess acetyl CoA is converted into acetoacetyl CoA. This then becomes acetoacetate in the liver, and finally acetone and β-hydroxybutyrate in the circulation. These end products are known as ketone bodies, and are important as a metabolic fuel for diabetics. However, if their rate of production exceeds the rate of usage, ketones accumulate in the blood stream leading to a ketosis.

Most of the H^+ ions from acetoacetate and β-hydroxybutyrate are buffered in the circulation, but severe metabolic acidosis can still arise. The low pH from an increase in acid leads to deep, rapid breathing known as Kussmaul breathing. Other effects of the acidosis include:
- Acidic urine, which cannot be buffered leading to ion loss, subsequent water loss and thus dehydration, hypotension and hypovolaemia.
- Acidosis and dehydration leading to coma (serious emergency). Coma can also be caused by hyperosmolarity with increased glucose concentration, lactate accumulation (lactic acidosis) and brain oedema.
- Severe acidosis coupled to a marked depletion of sodium ions, and high potassium since insulin is required to drive K^+ ions into cells.

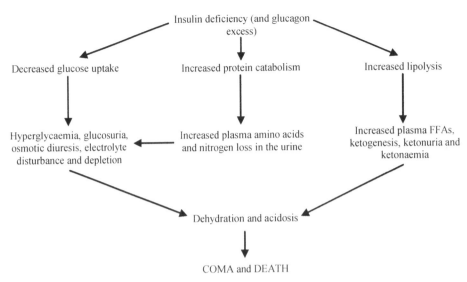

Figure 13.3 – Consequences of insulin deficiency

13.2.2 Diagnosis of Diabetes

In diabetes, glucose builds up in the bloodstream, especially after meals. Thus, to diagnose diabetes, it is possible to give an oral glucose load and measure if the blood glucose rises to a greater peak and returns to normal levels more slowly than expected. This is known as the Oral Glucose Tolerance Test (OGTT).

The OGTT is performed after an overnight fast (or a fast of at least 4-5 hours), with the patient allowed only water during this period. A standard dose of 75g anhydrous glucose is dissolved in 250-350ml of water and given orally. The patient is then told to sit up or lie on their side to facilitate stomach emptying and blood samples are collected 2 hours after the load is given. These post-load samples are compared to pre-load levels.

Before the OGTT is started, medication such as corticosteroids must be stopped. In addition, vulnerable patients, such as those post-illness or trauma should not be tested.

		Fasting Glucose (mmol/L)	2 hours Post-load glucose (mmol/L)
Normal	Venous plasma	<7.8	<7.8
	Venous blood	<6.7	<6.7
	Capillary blood	<6.7	<7.8
Diabetic	Venous plasma	>7.8	>11.1
	Venous blood	>6.7	>10.0
	Capillary blood	>6.7	>11.1

13.2.3 Principles of Treatment and Measurement of Control

Type 1
Many regimens are available for the treatment of type 1 diabetes depending on what is most suitable and convenient for the patient. The classic treatment regimen involves administering a dose of insulin just before or just after meals and snacks, in an attempt to mimic the controlled release of insulin from

130

the pancreas. Diabetics must monitor their blood glucose, and give doses on the basis of their prevailing levels, ensuring the correct amount is administered and complications are reduced.

Long-term measurement of control can be achieved in three ways:
1. HbA1c – haemoglobin undergoes non-enzymatic glycosylation over a long period of time. The extent of glycosylation to HbA1c depends on the average glucose over time. Thus, measurement of HbA1c levels gives an indication of the average blood glucose level over 1-2 months, since the half-life of HbA1c is around 60 days.
2. Glycosylated plasma proteins – measurement of glycosylated proteins such as albumin gives an indication of control over 10-15 days, since the half-life is shorter than Hb. This is particularly useful in maintaining tight control, such as in pregnant women.
3. Microalbuminuria – urinary loss of small amounts of albumin (microalbuminuria) can be detected by urine dipstick test, and is used to indicate the chance of progression to nephropathy (which occurs in 50% of diabetic patients).

Type 2
In type 2 diabetes, insulin is often not useful given the pathogenesis of the disease. Therefore other approaches are taken:
- Diet – reduce body weight, improving sensitivity of cells to insulin. Especially diets rich in complex carbohydrates to slow glucose absorption.
- Drugs
  - Sulphonylureas – inhibit K+ channels and so increase insulin release. Can induce hypoglycaemia.
  - Biguanides e.g. metformin – improve sensitivity to insulin and decrease appetite. Associated with anorexia, epigastric discomfort and diarrhoea.
  - Thiazolidinediones (glitazones) – reduce insulin resistance by interaction with peroxisome proliferators-activated receptor-γ (regulation of genes involved in lipid metabolism and insulin action).
  - α-glucosidase inhibitors – slow carbohydrate digestion and uptake .
- Newer drugs include repaglinide (insulin secretanalogue) and orlistat (inhibits lipase and so decreases fat absorption).

In the later stages of the disease, pancreatic amyloid formation and islet destruction occurs. As such, insulin treatment may be necessary.

13.2.4 Complications of Diabetes
The complications of diabetes can be divided into acute and chronic problems. The acute complications are described above, and include:
- Hypoglycaemia in insulin overdose – leads to sweating, pallor, tremor and an aggressive nature.
- Hyperglycaemia – see above.
- Diabetic ketoacidosis – see above.
- HONK – hyperosmolar non-ketotic acidosis, which can result in coma in type 2 diabetic.

The long-term complications of diabetes can be generally divided into those caused by microvascular, macrovascular and neurological changes. These can occur in almost all organs of the body. Some specific examples include:
- Macrovascular – the development of atherosclerosis
  - Stroke twice as likely.
  - MI three to five times as likely.

- - Amputation of foot from gangrene fifty times as likely.
    - Intensive treatment only has a small effect on cardiovascular risk.
  - Microvascular
    - Capillary abnormalities due to high glucose levels – abnormal protein glycosylation and the production of sorbitol leading to osmotic damage.
    - Retinopathy leading to blindness.
    - Neuropathy – nerve damage causing impotence, loss of bowel control and loss of sensation in the periphery.
    - Nephropathy, with small vessel changes leading to kidney failure. Treated with ACE inhibitors.
  - Neurological
    - Via vascular damage and also directly.
    - Symmetrical sensory polyneuropathy ('glove and stocking' distribution of sensory changes).
    - Ocular palsies.
    - Painful neuropathy.
    - Impotence and incontinence.
    - Postural hypotension due to damage to autonomic nerves.
    - Can have 'silent MIs' due to loss of sensation, such that patient is not aware of the pain from their heart attack.
  - Eye disease
    - Cataracts.
    - Neovascularisation leading to glaucoma.
  - Diabetic foot – ulcers can develop due to neuropathy, microvascular and macrovascular changes.
  - Susceptibility to infection, and injuries take longer to heal (due to protein depletion and high glucose culture medium) causing diabetic ulceration.

CHAPTER 14

Structure and Function of Genes

14.1 WHAT GENES DO

Genes are the physical and functional unit of heredity, which carry information from one generation to the next. Molecularly, they are defined as the entire nucleic acid sequence required for the synthesis of a functional polypeptide, including exons, introns and non-coding transcription control regions. At a gross level, genes define a certain phenotype, such as a physical characteristic. Genes encode for proteins, in addition to specialised RNA molecules such as tRNA and rRNA.

Mutations are permanent, hereditable changes in the nucleotide sequence of a chromosome, normally in a single gene. They commonly lead to the change or loss in normal function of the gene product or products. There are various types of mutation:

- Silent – harmless mutation in which the amino acid sequence is unchanged since the nucleotide change occurs at a degenerate position (e.g. both GGA and GGG code for glycine).
- Mis-sense – amino acid changing, can cause a damaging alteration in phenotype.
- Frame shift – insertion or deletion of base pairs leading to alterations in the codon sequence and thus catastrophic effects for gene product function.
- Non-sense – generation of a stop codon, which may also cause disease.

14.2 WHAT GENES ARE MADE OF

Genes are sequences of nucleic acid, consisting of 3-base codons, each of which codes for a particular amino acid. Each 3-base codon is composed from four bases – A, T, G and C (see later).

It was originally believed that proteins occupied the role of containing genetic information, but it was subsequently shown to be contained within DNA and RNA sequences.

14.3 CONNECTION BETWEEN GENE STRUCTURE AND FUNCTION

14.3.1 DNA structure and function

14.3.1.1 DNA structure
DNA is a long linear polymer, composed of nucleotide residues which, in its native state, arranges into a characteristic double helix. This double helix composes two antiparallel strands held together by hydrogen bonds between complimentary base pairs.

The four nucleotides that make up DNA have a common structure of a phosphate group linked by a phosphodiester bond to a pentose sugar (deoxyribose) linked to a base. In contrast, nucleosides are the combination of base and sugar only.

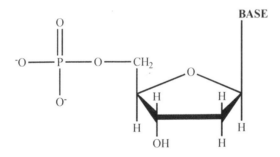

Figure 14.1 – Nucleotide structure

The four nucleotides are divided into the purines (two rings) and pyrimidines (one ring)
- Purines – adenine, guanine
- Pyramidines – cytosine, thymine (uracil in RNA)

In the DNA polynucleotide, the nucleotides are joined by 3'5'-phosphodiester bonds, forming a long chain. Each DNA stand has a 5' and 3' end, with the two complimentary strands making up the double helix running in opposite directions (i.e. 5' to 3' matched with 3' to 5'). The two complimentary strands are held together by numerous hydrogen bonds between the bases. Adenine and thymine are paired together, and interact via two hydrogen bonds. Guanine and cytosine are held together by three hydrogen bonds. There is no mixing of the base interactions i.e. guanine cannot bond with adenine due to the shape and size of each nucleotide.

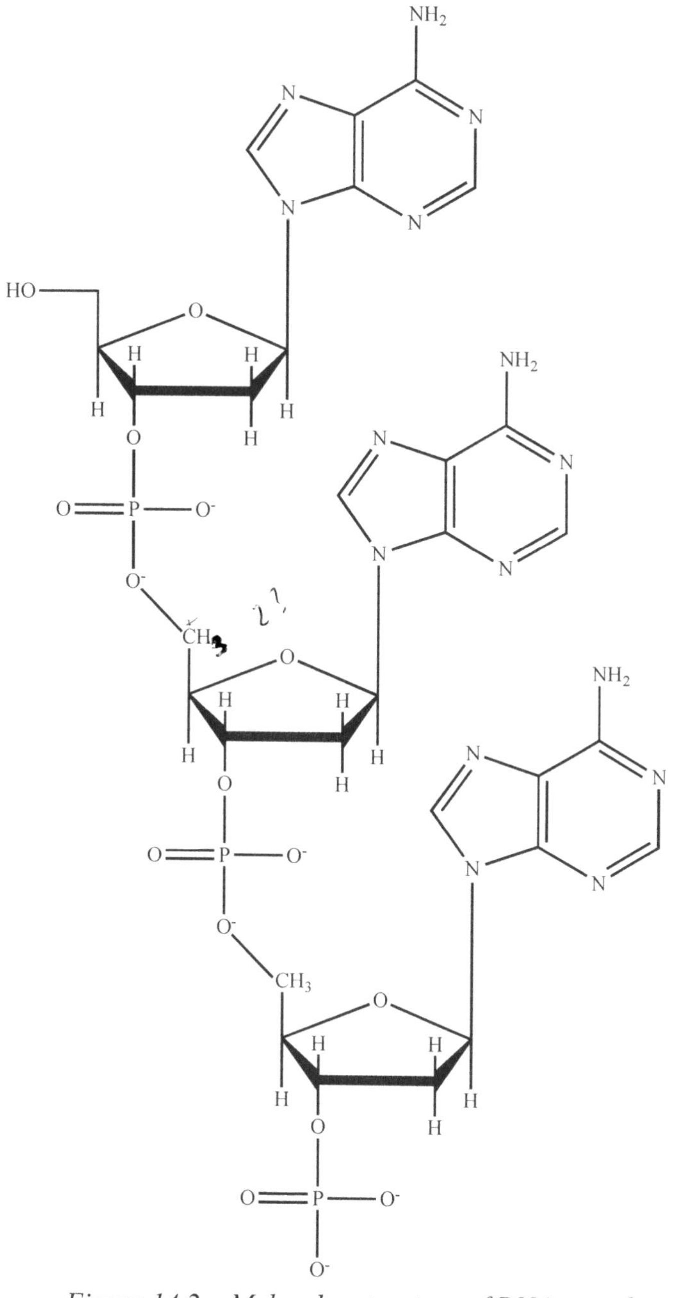

Figure 14.2 – Molecular structure of DNA strand

There is a plethora of experimental evidence for the existence of DNA as a helix. Firstly, DNA exists in an aqueous environment, yet all bases are hydrophobic with polar phosphates at the opposite end. Thus, arrangement as a helix allows the bases to be shielded from the aqueous environment, whilst exposing the phosphate groups. Secondly, stoichiometric analysis demonstrates A:T and G:C are present in equal ratios. This suggests these bases are paired, and since hydrogen bonding exists readily in water, the bonding of pyramidines and purines in this way is most appropriate. Finally, X-ray diffraction imagery (as used in the original work by Franklin, Watson and Crick) shows repeating helical structures.

135

14.3.1.2 The double helix

The double helix of DNA forms with the orientation of the two antiparallel strands such that the complimentary bases undergo bonding. This naturally forms a neat double helix with the maximum number of possible H-bonds to increase stability.

The double helix is right-handed, but not regular. There are major and minor grooves, important for the interaction of proteins during DNA replication and gene expression.

14.3.1.2 Importance of DNA structure

As a consequence of the arrangement of DNA into a double helix, negative charges on the external phosphates must be neutralised by histone proteins. This allows control of gene expression via alteration of these histone-DNA interactions. In addition, to read the base sequence, access to the inside of the molecule must be achieved, normally through interactions with the major groove – this provides the need for specific adaptations for DNA replication and gene expression.

Being complimentary, the two strands that make up the DNA double helix permit reading, repair and duplication from one generation to another. This arrangement and function is pivotal to normal cell function.

Separation of the DNA double helix can be achieved by heating a sample. This may result in denaturation and the formation of random structures. However, by gentle treatment, the nucleotide sequence of each strand can be maintained. Furthermore, lowering temperatures or increasing ion concentrations induces two DNA strands to re-associate. This forms the basis of hybridisation techniques used to assess the similarity of two DNA samples, and the isolation of a specific DNA sequence from a mixture of genes, fragments or larger stretches.

14.3.2 DNA replication

All organisms must replicate their DNA before cell division. This process is achieved by interaction of DNA with a number of proteins, and occurs at a rate of around 50 nucleotides per second in mammals.

DNA replication is a semi-conservative process. This describes the fact that each strand of the double helix is paired with a new strand in replication (i.e. each strand acts as a template for the formation of the new strand).

Meselson and Stahl demonstrated the semi-conservative nature of DNA replication using ^{15}N, which is incorporated into newly synthesising DNA. Replication of DNA solely in the presence of this nitrogen isotope leads to all DNA strands possessing 100% ^{15}N in the bases. Subsequent transfer of ^{15}N strand DNA to ^{14}N solution allows replication in the presence of this different isotope, and collection of the newly synthesised DNA. Centrifuge and density gradient analysis demonstrated all DNA strands were now a 50:50 mixture of ^{14}N and ^{15}N – thus each ^{15}N strand had been used as a template for the synthesis of a complimentary ^{14}N strand. Subsequent replication of these DNA samples in ^{14}N solution leads to half the samples being ^{14}N-^{15}N mixes, whilst the other half are 100% ^{14}N.

14.3.2.1 Origins and DNA polymerase

Replication of DNA starts at particular points in the sequence, which are recognised by binding proteins which may subsequently recruit polymerase enzymes. These regions of DNA are known as origins. At the origin, the double helix uncoils, allowing for bi-directional replication. This forms a 'replication bubble' consisting of two replication forks moving in opposite directions. Prokaryotes have circular chromosomes, and only one origin of replication, whilst eukaryotes have larger linear chromosomes, and thus use multiple origins of replication. Multiple origins allow rapid replication of DNA. Eventually the segments that have been replicated at each of the origins merge to produce a single, complete DNA strand.

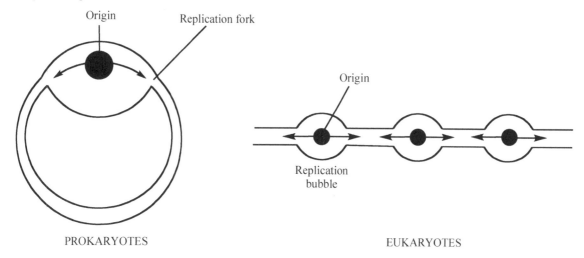

Figure 14.3 – Circular DNA replication and replication bubbles

Synthesis of new strands of DNA is performed by DNA polymerase. This enzyme catalyses the step-wise addition of nucleotides to the 3'-OH end of a growing strand, thus leading to synthesis in the 5' to 3' direction. dNTPs (forms of the four different nucleotides which may be added to the strand i.e. dATP, dGTP etc.) plus magnesium ions are required for the polymerisation reaction to occur, in which a phosphodiester bond is formed, releasing PP_i.

$$(DNA)_n + dNTP \rightarrow (DNA)_{n+1} + PP_i$$

DNA polymerase requires a template from which to copy (i.e. the existing strand) since there is only one active site present to bind to the dNTP. Thus, the dNTP that binds is determined by the base sequence of the template.

DNA polymerase is generally fast and accurate, however there are some limitations to its operation requiring adaptations to overcome these problems:
- Unable to unwind the DNA helix itself and separate the two strands.
- Unable to initiate a chain and therefore requires a DNA or RNA primer.
- Only able to operate in the 5' to 3' direction, leading to problems replicating one of the complimentary strands.

14.3.2.2 Process of replication and adaptations
1. Initiation
    - DNA polymerase is unable to break hydrogen bonds, and thus multimeric origin binding proteins play a key role in the assembly of the polymerase complex, and attraction of other enzymes to the region.
    - Helicases are attracted to the origin region, and move along the DNA strand, using ATP to separate the two parts of the helix.

- DNA is maintained in an unwound state (given the natural tendency for the strands to re-associate) by single stranded binding protein, which also acts to recruit DNA polymerase to the origin sites on both template strands.

2. Prevention of supercoiling
   - DNA helicase introduces supercoils into the DNA molecule when it separates the two strands.
   - To prevent this, DNA gyrase introduces right-handed supercoils into the helix during synthesis, which reverses the left-handed supercoils of DNA helicase.
   - In addition, topoisomerases break phosphodiester bonds between bases, allowing free rotation of DNA strands.

3. Priming
   - Short RNA sequences complimentary to the template strand (synthesised by RNA polymerase primase) bind to each of the two strands, allowing recruitment of high-fidelity DNA polymerase.
   - After DNA elongation, DNA polymerase I uses 5' to 3' exonuclease activity to remove the primer from the strand.

4. Strand synthesis
   - DNA replication occurs in both directions, outwards from the origin, forming two replication forks.
   - New DNA is synthesised against the template strand.

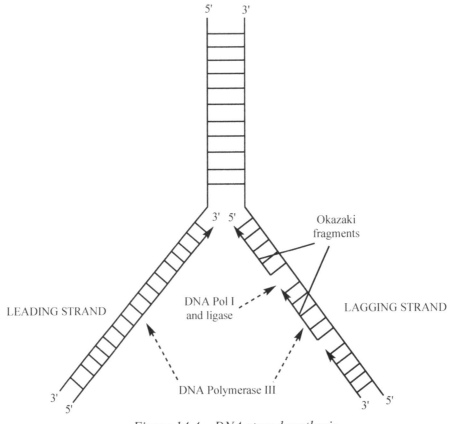

Figure 14.4 – DNA strand synthesis

- DNA polymerase is only able to elongate strands in the 5' to 3' direction – on the leading strand (3' to 5' template side of the original double helix) this causes no problem, and synthesis occurs in one go. On the lagging strand (5' to 3' template), synthesis occurs in fragments, known as Okazaki fragments, which must later be joined.
- Two forms of DNA polymerase are used during strand synthesis – DNA Pol III is used for the synthesis of the leading and lagging strand copies since it is rapid and accurate. DNA Pol I however acts as a gap filler for the lagging strand, removes primers via exonuclease activity and also synthesises the stretch of DNA previously occupied by the primers.
- Once the new strand has been synthesised, DNA ligase joins adjacent complimentary strands.

5. Telomere synthesis
- Due to the linear nature of mammalian chromosomes, the lagging strands would get shorter during each round of replication since there are terminal regions which cannot be copied by DNA polymerase.
- To prevent this, chromosomes have G-rich ends known as telomeres, which are re-synthesised during each round of replication by telomerase.
- This enzyme has its own in-built template and can thus prevent shortening.
- Shortening of telomeres is believed to be the molecular basis for ageing, whilst overactive telomerase can be important in cancer pathogenesis.

6. Proof reading and repair
- DNA polymerase I and III make mistakes (rarely).
- Both enzymes possess 3' to 5' exonuclease activity, which allows editing function during polymerisation.
- When an incorrect base is recognised, the exonuclease removes it and allows DNA Pol to return to this early position and insert the correct nucleotide.
- Other repair mechanisms include:
    - Base excision repair – removal of small areas of incorrect bases.
    - Nucleotide excision repair – removal of helix-distorting lesions by unravelling, removing and re-synthesising.
    - Double strand break repair by joining the ends of DNA fragments.
- Repair is particularly important in the prevention of oncogenic mutations, in addition to cell cycle control halting replication of damaged cells e.g. p53.

14.4 THE GENETIC CODE

In humans, 20 amino acids are encoded by 61 mRNA 3-base codons. This means the genetic code is degenerate (more than one codon for each amino acid). The code is read in a 5' to 3' direction. Four of the codon sequences are specialised to act as start and stop signals (note U is the mRNA equivalent of T):
- Start – AUG
- Stop – UAA, UAG, UGA

Due to the 3-base codon nature of the genetic code, there are three possible reading frames for a stretch of DNA, each one base along from the next. Thus, there is potential to encode very different polypeptides with the same genetic code.

14.5 tRNAs

Transfer RNAs provide adapter function, linking individual amino acids to each codon within the mRNA sequence. These molecules are synthesised by aminoacyl-tRNA synthase, making it an essential enzyme for protein synthesis.

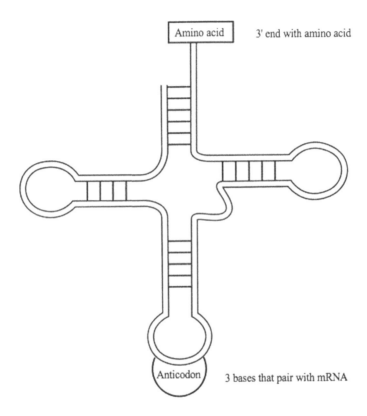

Figure 14.5 – tRNA structure

CHAPTER 15

The Regulation of Gene Expression

15.1 REGULATION OF GENE EXPRESSION
The regulation of expression of genes in all organisms is essential to their successful survival and replication. The approaches used by prokaryotes and eukaryotes vary, often reflecting the differing needs of each group of organisms. Structural genes (those which produce all proteins other than those involved in regulation e.g. enzymes, cytoskeletal elements) are controlled by the action of regulatory gene products (protein or RNA molecules involved in the regulation of one or more other genes).

15.2 REGULATION OF GENE EXPRESSION BY PROKARYOTES
Bacteria contain a small, condensed genome in a single circular chromosome. They have no control over the external environment, and therefore need to respond to stimuli as to use energy (and transcribe genes) when most appropriate.

The key unit of expression in bacteria is the operon. This is a group of genes that encodes proteins with related functions, and are expressed by being transcribed into a polycistronic mRNA molecule. Prokaryotic mRNA requires little or no processing before translation, with many being translated before transcription is even complete.

15.2.1 Stages of gene transcription

1. Initiation
   - RNA polymerase holoenzyme recognises specific promoter sites 10 to 35 bases upstream of the gene to be transcribed.
   - Promoter regions trigger the transcription initiation process, and thus genes with strong promoters are more frequently transcribed.
   - No primer required.
   - RNA Pol is able to unwind DNA helix itself, locally exposing a single stranded template.

2. Elongation
   - One subunit of the RNA polymerase holoenzyme dissociates, allowing elongation to be carried out by the core enzyme – this moves along the antisense strand, synthesising a complimentary strand using ribonucleotide 5'triphosphates as precursors.
   - DNA rewinds once transcription is complete.

3. Termination
   - RNA Pol encounters a termination sequence (GC rich then AT rich region), which synthesises a self-complimentary portion of RNA. This forms a hairpin loop, which acts as a block to transcription.
   - Also, Rho protein termination factor can be involved – recognises specific sequence on nascent RNA, causing RNA to wrap around the hexameric protein which then detaches RNA from DNA using helicase activity. If Rho protein catches up with RNA polymerase, then termination occurs.

15.2.2 Control of gene expression – response to external stimuli

15.2.2.1 The bacterial operon

Bacterial genes encoding proteins with related functions may be organised into clusters, allowing transcription of polycistronic mRNA from a single promoter. Thus, control of a single promoter can regulate the activity of an entire pathway. The unit of expression – the operon – is either inducible or repressible, with gene expression regulated at the level of transcription to prevent energy wastage.

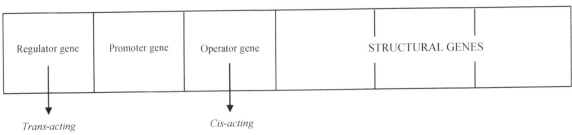

Figure 15.1 – Bacterial operon

15.2.2.2 The lac operon – negative control

The lac operon was discovered by Jacob and Monod. It is an operon employed by bacteria, including E. coli. It ensures that when organisms are grown in glucose containing medium, enzymes for lactose metabolism are present at a low concentration, whilst growth in lactose containing medium induces their expression.

When lactose is added to a medium containing bacteria, three enzymes are induced:
- Z – β-galactosidase, which hydrolyses lactose to glucose and galactose.
- Y – lactose permease, which transports lactose across the bacterial cell wall.
- A – transacetylase, with poorly understood function.

Initially, the amount of enzyme induced was found to be proportional to the concentration of medium used. Thus, Jacob and Monod deduced that the rate of synthesis of all three gene products was controlled by a common regulatory product, which binds to the lac operon to prevent transcription. Furthermore, mutants in which the lacI gene was knocked out (lacI produces a repressor protein) were constitutively active, and produced all three enzymes in equal proportion, demonstrating common control under one promoter.

When no lactose is present, the regulator region of the lac operon produces a repressor protein which, by binding to the operator stretch of the operon, is able to prevent Z, Y and A gene transcription. Thus, this is an example of negative control. When lactose is present however, it enters the cell and binds to the lac repressor protein. This decreases the affinity of the repressor for its binding site, thus allowing the initiation of transcription of the operon and enzyme synthesis.

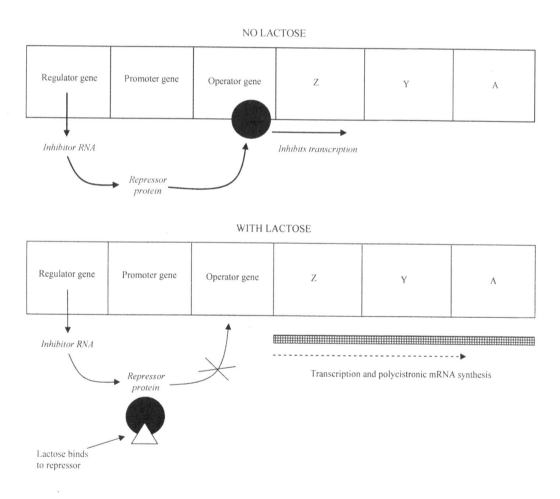

Figure 15.2 – The lac operon

15.2.2.3 Catabolite gene activation – positive control
Glucose is the preferential substrate for E. coli, and can be used directly by the cell without enzyme induction. However, when glucose levels fall, other substrates must be used instead, and thus there is positive control working in conjunction with the lac operon to ensure this occurs.

Upstream of the lac operon promoter is another region which binds catabolic activating protein (CAP). This induces the binding of RNA polymerase, and thus the transcription of lac operon enzymes. CAP can only bind to DNA when complexed with cAMP (which acts as an energy signal of the cell since adenylate cyclase is inhibited by glucose). Thus, when glucose and ATP levels fall, cAMP levels increase, increasing the level of CAP-cAMP complex and thus the transcription of the lac operon structural genes. Working in conjunction with the negative control described above, this gives an added level of control.

15.2.2.4 The trp operon
The trp operon encodes 5 enzymes in E. coli that synthesise tryptophan. These are synthesised co-ordinately and in equimolar amounts since they are derived from a single polycistronic mRNA. Trp mRNA has a short half-life however, allowing bacteria to respond rapidly to changes in extracellular tryptophan, under the control of the trp repressor.

Experimentally, deletion of a region between the operator and structural stretches of DNA in E. coli leads to an increase in mRNA. This demonstrated another gene – known as the leader peptide sequence – was present in this gap. It was later shown that the leader peptide sequence encodes for, amongst other amino acids, two tryptophan residues.

In the trp operon, translation occurs with transcription – RNA polymerase starts transcribing, and then pauses to allow ribosomes to translate the leader peptide sequence. If tryptophan levels are low, translation pauses at the two tryptophan codons, and the ribosome inhibits the formation of a termination hairpin. This thus allows synthesis of the structural genes, and subsequently tryptophan-synthesising enzymes. When tryptophan levels are high, however, the entire leader peptide is synthesised, inducing the formation of a termination hairpin which prevents RNA Pol I from enzyme translation.

15.2.2.5 DNA inversions in Salmonella
Flagellae are long, thin helical proteins that allow Salmonella and other organisms to move in the intestine. Salmonella have two genes for flagellin proteins (from which flagella are constructed) known as H1 and H2. Only one of these genes is expressed at any one time. Random switching between H1 and H2 allows the bacteria to evade the host immune response, which is targeted at flagellin proteins.

mRNA for H1 is also the template for the H2 repressor and vice versa. Thus, when H1 is produced, the H2 promoter and H1 repressor are both inactive. This relies on an inversion of the DNA, which allows the transcription of either H1 or H2 depending on the orientation of the DNA. DNA inversion is performed by a recombinase enzyme, which catalyses the cleavage and strand exchange required for switching of the chosen flagellin protein. It is thought this process occurs regularly and randomly, such that the host immune system is constantly 'chasing' the bacteria.

15.3 REGULATION OF GENE EXPRESSION BY EUKARYOTES
In eukaryotes, the regulation of tissue specific gene expression is essential for:
  -   Cell differentiation.
  -   Varying activity of enzymes, such as those in glycolysis.

GLUCOSE, LOW cAMP, NO LACTOSE

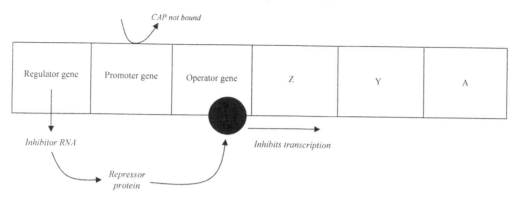

GLUCOSE, LOW cAMP, HIGH LACTOSE

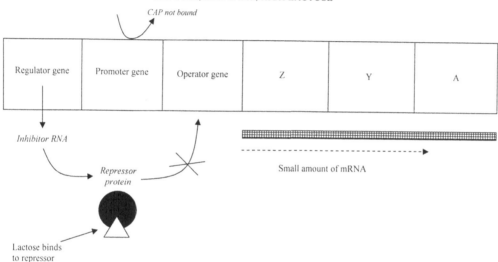

LOW GLUCOSE, HIGH cAMP, HIGH LACTOSE

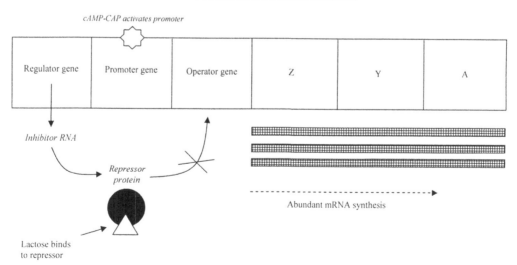

Figure 15.3 – CAP operon

- Determination of cell fate and function.
- Change in expression over time e.g. during development in response to stimuli such as hormones, to ensure gene activation when required.

Gene expression can theoretically be controlled at all levels, but the majority of it occurs at transcription to ensure no superfluous intermediates are synthesised.

Typically, each gene has several regulatory elements and is under the control of many trans-acting transcription factors. These interact with each other and other proteins in the transcription initiation complex to increase or decrease the rate of transcription.

15.3.1 RNA polymerase enzymes
The nucleus of eukaryotic cells has three types of RNA polymerase:
- RNA Pol I – rRNA synthesis in the nucleolus.
- RNA Pol II – mRNA synthesis of both housekeeping and tissue specific genes.
- RNA Pol III – small RNA synthesis e.g. tRNA, snRNA.

Transcription by large, multi-subunit RNA Pol II involves three stages:
- Initiation of synthesis.
- Elongation of the strand.
- Termination of transcription at certain positions downstream of the gene.

The result of transcription is a complimentary primary transcript, which can be modified to form a final mRNA transcript from which polypeptides can be synthesised.

The regulation of transcription occurs at a number of stages:
- Formation of the transcription initiation complex.
- Activation of the gene to be transcribed by changes in chromatin structure.
- Control of the levels and activity of transcription factors within the cell.

15.3.2 Initiation of transcription
RNA Pol II usually starts transcription of a gene at a specific site on the DNA template, just upstream of the protein coding region. The start sites can be identified using labelled nascent transcripts or more precisely by primer extension.

Core promoter elements
- Defined as the minimal DNA sequence necessary for the accurate transcription of a gene by RNA Pol II.
- Most common CPE is the TATA box sequence, located 30-35bp upstream of the start site – a single point mutation in the TATA box sequence has been shown to drastically decrease the transcription of the adjacent gene.
- In some eukaryotic cells the 'initiator element' is used.
- When neither TATA box nor initiator is present, initiation may occur at CpG islands, located over a 200bp stretch.

General transcription factors
- Even the strongest of CPE is unable to induce Pol II to transcribe without the activity of ancillary factors – shown in 1979 that the activity of pure RNA Pol II for in vitro gene expression when added to crude cell extract was negligible.
- 6 general transcription factors have been identified, which must assemble on the promoter region before Pol II can bind and start transcription.

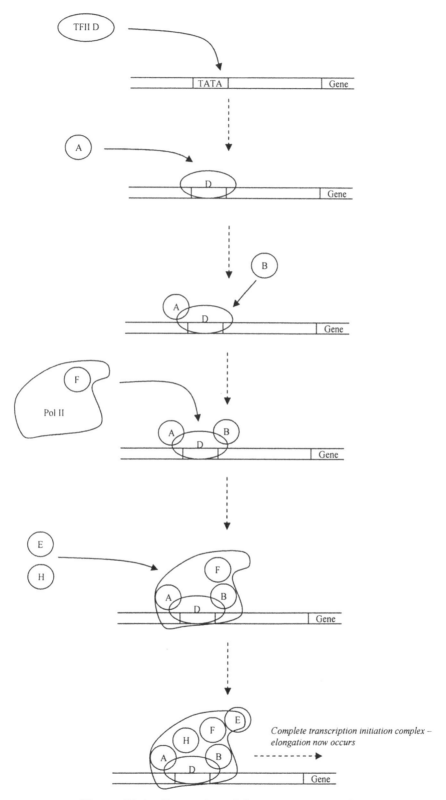

Figure 15.4 – Formation of the initiation complex

15.3.2.1 Regulation of transcription initiation

Typically, each gene is controlled by several trans-factors which bind to cis-elements. The trans-factors interact with each other and with general transcription factors to regulate the rate of formation of the transcription initiation complex (TIC) and hence the rate of transcription of that gene.

Cis-acting factors

Promoter proximal elements

- Regulator elements 100-200bp upstream of the promoter.
- When individual base substitutions are introduced into the region 100bp upstream of the β-globin gene start point, it was found to induce downregulation when the mutations were present in the TATA box, CAAT box and GC box regions (both upstream proximal promoter elements).

Enhancers

- Additional regulatory sequences located thousands of base pairs upstream or downstream of the transcription sites, within the gene itself or in an intron region.
- Shown that when the enhancer region of the SV40 genome was added to a β-globin gene, it stimulated transcription 100-fold, even when distant from the initiator region of the gene.
- Orientation independent.
- Commonly believed to influence the promoter region by folding:

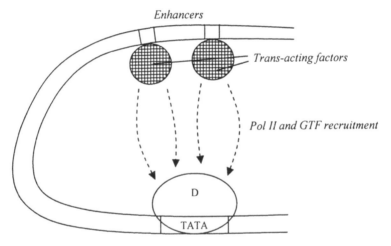

Figure 15.5 – Enhancer function

Locus control regions

- These are similar to enhancers, but limited by their orientation and distance.
- Thought to work by establishing an 'open' chromatin conformation, which inhibits the normal repression of transcription over an area spanning several genes.

Trans-acting factors

Trans-acting sequence specific factors bind to cis-acting regulatory sequences and mediate their effects. It is estimated that 10% of the human genome encodes for these factors, which may be activating or repressing.

Crucial to their function, trans-acting factors have two functional domains:
- DNA binding domain – interacts with specific sequences of DNA via structural motifs such as helix-loop-helix regions and zinc fingers.
- Activation domain – interacts with other proteins, stimulating transcription from the nearby promoter region e.g. acidic, glutamine rich and proline rich domains.

Co-ordinate control is employed by trans-acting factors. Thus, a single activator may be used to activate multiple genes allowing co-ordinated transcription, or a number of activators may be required for one gene to be transcribed. This is known as combinatorial control. An example of this is the transthyretin gene, controlled by more than 5 transcription factors, all of which must be present for transcription to occur.

The binding of multiple transcriptional regulators to sites on enhancer DNA forms enhanceosomes. This has several advantages for gene activation, since it means that low concentrations of transcription factors are capable of a large range of transcriptional activations through combinatorial control. In addition, this enables integration of multiple regulatory 'inputs' into a single 'output'.

Transcriptional repressors are much less common than activators. They can act through direct interference with the function of activators, the formation of a non-DNA binding complex with activators or by masking the activation domain. It has been shown that designated repressor proteins do exist, mutations in which lead to increased gene expression. For example, the Wilm's tumour in children is related to a lack of WT1 repressor protein, which inhibits EGRI. WT1 is likely to interfere with transcriptional activation.

The role of chromatin
In vitro, all DNA is accessible to transcription factors and initiation complex proteins. However, in vivo, DNA is organised into nucleosomes, suggesting that its recognition by RNA Pol II is subject to different constraints.

Typically, the organisation of eukaryotic chromatin provides a barrier to transcription since it prevents transcriptional machinery from interacting with promoter DNA. There are two methods of chromatin remodelling which play an important part in gene regulation:
- Covalent modification of histones – acetylation, methylation, phosphorylation and ubiquitination. This allows a 'histone code' of covalent modifications. It is believed that covalent modification alters the affinity of DNA for histone proteins, thus altering the conformation of the nucleosome and increasing the accessibility of the DNA.
- Chromatin remodelling complexes – examples include the swi/snf complex, which is ATP dependent and can cause a conformational change in the chromatin structure.

Regulation of transcription factor levels
Regulation can involve the stable, long-term change in the expression of transcription factors in response to multiple regulatory interactions, such as during development. Examples of this include the action of steroid hormones, inducing their long-term effects:
1. Steroid hormone diffuses into cell.
2. Interacts with (often cytoplasmic) receptor element and dimerises.
3. Enter the nucleus.
4. Binds to the hormone response element upstream of a gene.
5. Induces gene-specific transcription.

15.3.2.2 Transcriptional elongation and termination

The majority of work into the function of Pol II transcription systems focuses on initiation. However, sites of regulation also exist in the elongation and termination stages.

The largest subunit of Pol II contains a unique CTD region. This may be phosphorylated (to induce elongation) or dephosphorylated (in the formation of the TIC). CTD phosphorylation also induces promoter clearance and the progression to the elongation phase of transcription. Furthermore, general transcription factor TFII S, and the factors elongin and ELL are also able to regulate the elongation phase.

Transcriptional termination is dependent on the presence of functional poly(A) signals at the 3' end of a transcript, and the sequences up and downstream of this poly(A) signal. There are two theories as to how termination arises. The anti-termination theory states that a conformational change in the transcriptional complex on recognising the poly(A) region leads to termination. The torpedo theory suggests that cleavage of the poly(A) site initiates termination through promotion of rapid degradation of the 3' product still associated with the elongating polymerase, thus detaching it from the mRNA transcript.

15.4 THE ROLE OF CHROMATIN

It is estimated that the human genome contains around 10^9 nucleotides, which would reach around 10 metres in length as extended DNA. This DNA must be compacted into a nucleus which is only 2μm in diameter – this is only possible through the characteristics of eukaryotic chromatin (a complex of DNA and the proteins – both histones and non-histones – to which it is bound).

It was originally assumed that chromatin had only a structural role, but it has been demonstrated that the expression of genes in higher organisms is acutely dependent on the accessibility of transcription factors, thus implicating chromatin organisation in the control of gene expression. Modifications affecting chromatin may be covalent or ATP-dependent.

The interaction and integration of such modification processes is responsible for the differential gene expression essential for the development, structure and function of eukaryotic cells.

15.4.1 Chromatin Structure

The basic structural unit of chromatin is the nucleosome. The nucleosome consists of 146 base pairs of DNA wrapped around a histone octamer core, containing two of each of the core histone proteins (H2A, H2B, H3 and H4). Strings of nucleosomes lead to the fundamental repeating unit of chromatin – nucleosome core followed by linker DNA and histone H1:

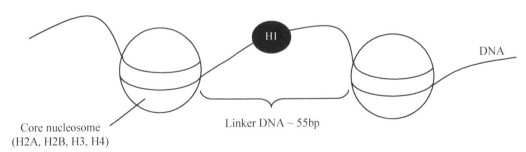

Figure 15.6 – Nucleosome structure

Subsequently, the string of nucleosomes with DNA wrapped around them may be organised into higher order structures, eventually giving rise to the condensed metaphase chromatin found in eukaryotic cells:

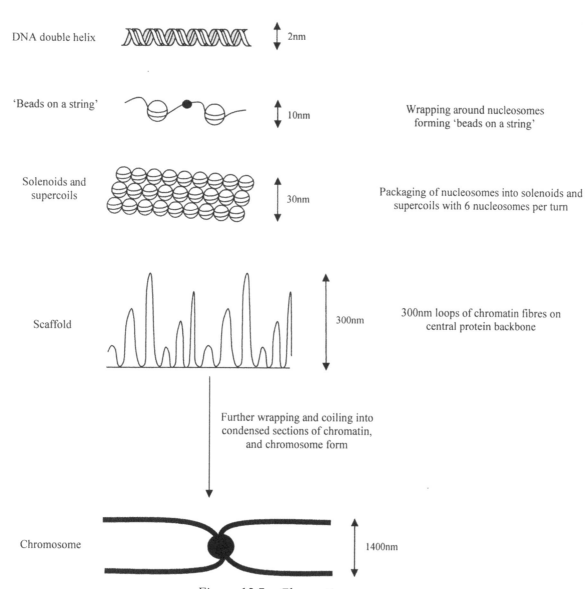

DNA double helix — 2nm

'Beads on a string' — 10nm — Wrapping around nucleosomes forming 'beads on a string'

Solenoids and supercoils — 30nm — Packaging of nucleosomes into solenoids and supercoils with 6 nucleosomes per turn

Scaffold — 300nm — 300nm loops of chromatin fibres on central protein backbone

Further wrapping and coiling into condensed sections of chromatin, and chromosome form

Chromosome — 1400nm

Figure 15.7 – Chromatin structure

What is known about the structure of chromatin has been largely learnt from study of metaphase (stage of mitosis in the eukaryotic cell cycle in which condensed chromosomes align along the centre of the cell), polytene (giant chromosomes formed when multiple rounds of replication produce many homologous chromatids that remain synapsed together, without cell division) and lampbrush chromosomes (large chromosomes found especially in the oocytes of amphibians, birds and other animals).

151

In addition, DNase I digestion experiments have demonstrated the break-down of chromatin into its individual histone octamer units, and then dissociation of histone proteins from the DNA using 6M urea. There is, however, a danger of artefaction in these experiments, suggesting density changes may merely be due to microscopy preparation.

15.4.2 Structure-Function Relationship and Regulation of Gene Transcription

The coiling of DNA around the histone octamer in the nucleosome is accepted to be the cornerstone of transcriptional control. One current theory suggests that nucleosomes suppress all genes, except for those whose transcription is brought about by specific positive regulatory components. Thus, nucleosomes effectively establish a baseline above which transcriptional and replicational control can be observed.

Nucleosomes are able to repress transcription in at least three different ways:
1. Occlude sites of protein-DNA binding and thus interfere with the interaction of activator and repressor proteins, polymerases and transcription factors.
2. Repress entire chromosome domains via higher order coiling of nucleosomes.
3. Repress gene expression in a hereditary manner, through the interaction of nucleosomes with additional chromosomal proteins in heterochromatin.

15.4.3 Experimental Evidence for the Importance of Chromatin Structure

The first indication of the variation in chromatin structure was demonstrated in the 1930's. Light microscopy distinguished two types of chromatin in the interphase nucleus – highly condensed heterochromatin and less condensed euchromatin.

Long before anything was known about the structure of chromatin, it was observed that individual chromosome bands in insect polytene chromosomes expanded and re-condensed. The changes in these bands coincided with the activation and silencing of genes within each region, suggesting a major change in DNA packaging accompanies gene activity.

In humans, the classic example of gene transcription alteration by changes in chromatin structure is demonstrated by X inactivation. In females, one copy of the X chromosome remains in the heterochromatin state (known as the Barr body), remaining transcriptionally inactive through many generations.

Later, nuclei isolated from vertebrate cells were exposed to increasing concentrations of the micrococcal endonuclease DNase I. DNA was subsequently isolated and Southern blotted, and it was found that 10% of the genome degraded preferentially under the influence of these enzymes. Also, the genes being degraded largely corresponded with those being expressed at the time. Even genes transcribed only a few times every generation were sensitive to DNase I, suggesting that a special state of chromatin, rather than DNA transcription itself made these regions particularly accessible for digestion.

Some sites within actively transcribed genes have been subsequently found to be hypersensitive to DNase, and thus demonstrated to be almost free of nucleosomes. This demonstrates that there is dynamic regulation of the structure of chromatin, with changes in the sensitivity to nucleases. It has been suggested that such hypersensitive sites are those associated with the enhancers and promoters required for eukaryotic gene expression.

Despite the obvious importance of chromatin structure in gene expression, only a small proportion of those genes contained within euchromatin are actively transcribed at any one point. Thus, while location within euchromatin is necessary for gene transcription, it is not sufficient, and other factors (e.g. transcription factors) are required.

15.4.4 Histone Modifications and Regulation

Each histone contains two domains – a histone fold, containing DNA in the central core particle, and a lysine rich N-terminal tail, which extends beyond the core particle. This tail provides a point of interaction for higher order coiling, condensation and many of the regulatory covalent modifications.

15.4.4.1 Acetylation

The original experiments which implicated acetylation in gene regulation noted that transcriptionally active cells were enriched with acetylated histone forms, whilst deacetylated histones were associated with transcriptional repression.

Acetylation occurs at condensed lysine residues on the amino acid terminal tails of core histones. Experiments in which these target lysines are mutated have been shown in yeast to alter the patterns of gene expression.

It has been suggested that acidic acetyl groups partially neutralise the basic nature of histones. This decreases their affinity for DNA, thus altering the nucleosome conformation and leading to an increased accessibility for transcriptional regulators to chromatin templates. Alternatively, acetylation may facilitate the binding of some transcription factors to the core promoter, or bring about the disruption of higher-order chromosome structure.

Histone acetylation is performed by histone acetyltransferase (HAT) enzymes. The first transcription-associated HAT was cloned by Brownell *et al.* in 1996, and since then many have been identified, such as Gcn5 in yeast and CBP, p300 in humans. It is thought that the largest subunit of the general transcription factor TFIID may function by acetylating the N-terminal tails of histones in the vicinity of the TATA box.

Histone deacetylation is performed by histone deacetylase (HDAC) enzymes. These are associated with transcriptional repression, and rather than binding specific sequences of DNA, associate with other chromatin proteins. Several nuclear repressor proteins (e.g. Ume6 in yeast, Mad/Max and Mxi/Max in mammals) interact with an HDAC containing the protein Sin3. Subsequently, this complex associates with another protein resulting in localised histone deacetylation and transcriptional repression. It is now clear that deacetylating histone proteins H3 and H4 allows access for other enzymes, which induces different covalent modifications in other lysine residues of their N-terminal tails.

Histone deacetylation also explains the observed correlation between DNA methylation and gene silencing. A protein that binds methylated DNA is able to recruit a multi-protein HDAC complex. This leads to the mechanism of genetic imprinting in which the expression level of a gene depends upon its parental origin, since DNA methylation (and thus the extent of acetylation and repression) is inherited.

15.4.4.2 Methylation

In recent years it has been shown that methylated histones play a role in the heterochromatic repression, promoter regulation and the propagation of the repressed state via DNA methylation. Many lysine methyltransferases have been identified, such as Suvar 39.
Methylation may act to stabilize the nucleosome, preventing transcription factors from binding and so inhibiting gene expression. It has also been suggested they may attract histone deacetylases, leading to histone deacetylation and gene repression.

15.4.4.3 Phosphorylation and Ubiquitination

Phosphorylation is a less well studied modification. It has a paradoxical role, being involved in the condensation of chromosomes during mitosis, but the opening of chromatin during transcriptional activation. There is also growing evidence that ubiquitination may be significant.

15.4.4.4 The Histone Code

'The histone code' describes the unifying concept that the combination of modifications, both in kind and number, dictate specific biological outcomes. The code is 'set' by histone-modifying enzymes of a defined specificity, and 'read' by non-histone proteins that bind in a modification-dependent way, giving rise to highly sensitive transcriptional control.

15.4.5 Chromatin Remodelling Complexes and Regulation

Chromatin remodelling complexes are multi-subunit structures which utilise ATP to remodel the nucleosomal structure and facilitate transcription. They do this by making chromatin more dynamic, catalysing the equilibrium between multiple structural states.

An important example of chromatin remodelling complexes is swi/snf and rsc complexes in yeasts. These are thought to act by facilitating an exchange between normal and more accessible chromatin conformations, thus providing an opportunity for transcription factors to bind to DNA. In the presence of purified swi/snf complex, nucleosomal DNA becomes more susceptible to DNase I digestion, suggesting its action involves a transient dissociation of DNA from the nucleosomal surface, possibly via a helicase-like action.

Recently, antibody-based studies have suggested that nucleosome remodelling and histone deacetylation activities exist in the same complex. This lends weight to the idea that HAT and HDAC activity may also be coupled to certain ATP-driven processes, and not just occur independently.

15.4.6 A Synthesised View and the Involvement of Transcription Factors

It has been suggested that transcriptional activators may bind promoters, recruiting chromatin-remodelling complexes and coordinating the assembly of the TIC. However, recent work has shown the system to be much more complex than this.

At the promoter of the yeast HO gene, swi/snf action controls the recruitment of HAT and subsequent chromatin remodelling. This governs the binding of an activator to the promoter. In the human IFN-β gene promoter, however, a virally induced HAT remodelling enzyme facilitates the movement of swi/snf, and thus drives the formation of the TIC on the gene promoter.

Many questions as to the role of chromatin, and how its structure is controlled remain unanswered.

15.4.7 Replication

The regulation of replication by chromatin structure follows similar principles to gene transcription. In order to be replicated, chromatin must be in a relaxed state. Blocks of heterochromatin have thus been found to replicate later than euchromatin (e.g. Barr body replicates much later than the other X chromosome in women). However, once initiation has occurred, replication moves at a similar rate in both heterochromatin and euchromatin. This suggests that the degree of chromatin condensation affects the order in which regions are initiated, and not the rate of movement of the replication fork. It has been suggested that transcription factors may bind to sequences adjacent to the replication origin, recruiting chromatin-remodelling complexes in order to create nucleosome-free regions and thus allow access of replication factors and activation of the origin.

15.4.8 RNAi and Chromatin

Recent evidence has shown that RNA interference may be core to chromatin regulation. RNA interference (RNAi) is a mechanism that inhibits gene expression by causing the degradation of specific RNA molecules or hindering the transcription of specific genes. RNAi targets include RNA from viruses and transposons (probably as a form of innate immune response), and also plays a role in regulating development and genome maintenance. It involves short RNA molecules complimentary to the target strand, and the RNA-induced silencing complex (RISC) which may induce breakdown or modification of the targeted strand.

Recently, RNAi machinery in *S. pombe* has been shown to be essential in the assembly of silent condensed chromatin at centrosomes and at the mating type region. Schramke *et al.* (2003) showed that previously euchromatic genes can be directly targeted by RNAi-dependent heterochromatin formation, and that this silencing pathway acts on endogenous repeats important in the determination of sex during the yeast sexual cycle.

The mechanism of RISC action is currently unknown, but thought to induce or recruit histone modification enzymes.

CHAPTER 16

RNA Processing and Translation

16.1 MRNA MODIFICATIONS

In eukaryotes, after transcription, the primary transcript must be modified before it can function as mRNA. This involves:
- 5' capping
- 3' polyadenylation and cleavage
- Splicing
- Further editing, methylation etc.

Considerable evidence suggests that these processes occur co-transcriptionally with trans-acting factors stimulating both modifications and mRNA synthesis. This has lead to the formation of the idea that the transcription and processing occur together in gene expression factories, which increase speed and efficiency.

16.1.1 5' Capping

Very soon after RNA Pol II starts making the transcript, and before RNA is more than 20-30 nucleotides long, the 5' end is chemically modified by the addition of a 7-methylguanosine residue in three steps:

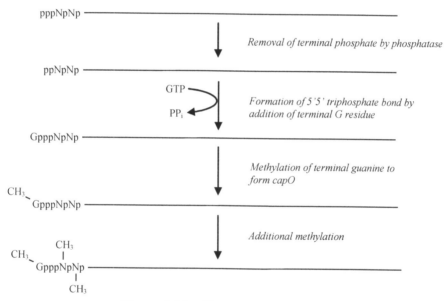

Figure 16.1 – Formation of the 5' cap

These caps are added in reverse polarity via a 5'5' triphosphate bridge, which forms a barrier to 5' exonucleases, and thus stabilises the transcript. The cap is also important for splicing, nuclear transport and translation. The cap is recognised by the cap binding complex (CBC) which is replaced by a translation factor on leaving the nuclear pore complex. This enhances translation in the cytoplasm.

16.1.2 3' Polyadenylation and cleavage

Almost all protein coding mRNAs (but not histone genes) contain a uniform 3' end consisting of up to 250 adenosine residues. The 3' end of the transcript is not defined by termination of transcription, but by the cleavage of the growing transcript and addition of a poly(A) tail. Thus, the poly(A) tail is not itself encoded by DNA.

Investigation in SV40 RNA shows adenosine residues are added to a 3' OH group created by cleavage. It has been shown that there is a AAUAAA sequence upstream of the poly(A) tail, and if this is mutated, polyadenylation does not occur leading to rapid degradation of the mRNA transcript. A GU or U-rich sequence downstream is also needed:

1. Cleavage and polyadenylation specificity factor (CPSF) forms a unstable complex with the AAUAAA region, attracting cleavage stimulatory factor I and II.
2. Cleavage stimulatory factor interacts with the GU/U region downstream, stabilising the complex.
3. Poly(A) polymerase enzyme binds to the complex, stimulating cleavage at the poly(A) site and releasing the cleavage factors. PAP adds adenosine residues slowly to the 3' ends as they are generated. This process can be accelerated by poly(A) binding protein II.
4. After 200-255 residues have been added, PABP II signals to PAP to stop polymerisation, with RNA Pol II continually transcribing and reaching termination at a later site.

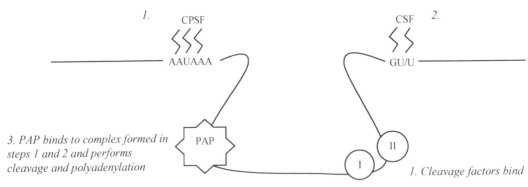

Figure 16.2 - Polyadenylation

The functions of the addition of a poly(A) tail include:
- Protection from degradation by nucleases.
- Termination of transcription due to a conformational change when cleavage factors leave.
- Aid for splicing – whether the poly(A) site is within an intron (and therefore is spliced out) or exon decides whether or not a protein is in the membrane or secreted form e.g. IgM in B-cells may act as either membrane-bound receptors or secreted antibodies depending on the spliced sequences.

16.1.3 Splicing
In 1977, it was discovered that eukaryotic genes are composed of alternative coding (exon) and non-coding (intron) sequences. This was demonstrated by electron microscopy of RNA-DNA hybrids between adenovirus DNA and the mRNA encoding a major protein in the adenovirus. This revealed that the RNAs were not entirely complimentary to the viral DNA with looping occurring. Each of these loops with no DNA-RNA interaction thus represents an intron.

Splicing is the process whereby introns may be removed and exon sequences joined together to form a mature mRNA sequence. Walter Gilbert suggested in 1978 that various combinations of exons could be spliced together to produce large numbers of different final mRNA molecules, representing isoforms of the same gene. This is known as alternative splicing and is important because it:
- Increases the diversity of protein production, explaining the complexity of the human body given a limited number of genes.
- Provides a mechanism for the regulation of gene expression.

The splicing mechanism:

1. Recognition of intron-exon boundary, marked by a moderately conserved short consensus sequence. This must be accurate since a single nucleotide slip in the splice point would shift the reading frame of the gene, and thus lead to an entirely different amino acid sequence. This is seen in some forms of thalassemia. Splicing will still occur effectively if exons from two different organisms are placed together.

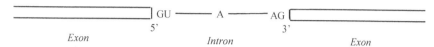

Figure 16.3 – Structure of intron-exon boundaries

2. Cleavage and transesterification – characterisation of mRNA that appears as intermediates during the splicing mechanism suggests two sequential transesterification reactions occur. The intron is looped round into a lasso structure, in which the intron is joined in an unusual 2'5' phosphodiester bond to an adenosine near the 3' end of the intron. The remaining exons can then be ligated:

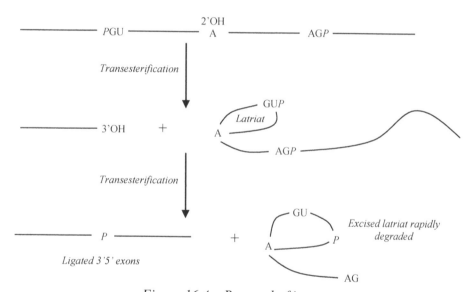

Figure 16.4 – Removal of introns

3. SnRNPs – these are complexes of proteins associated with a stable small RNA molecule, which interact with the RNA to form a spliceosome. The spliceosome is a catalytic assembly of proteins and RNA (consisting of over 200 factors) with U1, U2, U4, U5 and U6 snRNPs helping to form the final C complex that performs the splicing. This explains the need for the branch point (central A) and specific GU/AG sites, since snRNPs bind selectively to these sequences.

4. Exon definition – the average exon is 150 nucleotides long, while introns are 500 to 500,000 nucleotides long. Therefore, special machinery is required to recognise exons. Splicing factors bind to 3' and 5' splice sites across an exon (thus defining its position) before switching to interact with factors at the upstream 5' splice sites across the intron.

If the exon is greater than 300 nucleotides, it is not recognised. In very long introns, reversive splicing occurs where the inner portion of the intron are removed before total splicing:

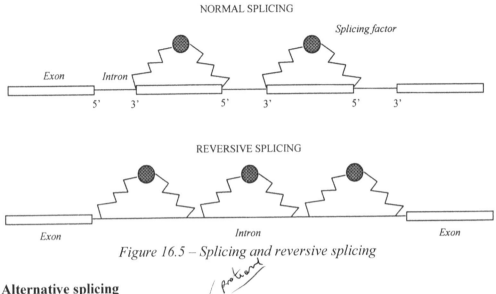

Figure 16.5 – Splicing and reversive splicing

16.1.4 Alternative splicing
Alternative splicing is the process by which multiple mRNAs are generated from the same pre-mRNA by differential joining of 3' and 5' splice sites. This explains how humans (with 32,000 genes) can have an increased complexity of proteosome compared to worms (with 19,000 genes) with only a small increase in genetic material. However, in protozoans, trans-splicing can occur where mRNA molecules are spliced together to generate variation.

Alternative splicing serves a role in development (sex determination), regulation and diversity. It is thought that as much as 50-60% of human genes have alternative splice forms such that a number of diseases (such as insulin-dependent diabetes mellitus and cancer) are associated with aberrant gene splicing.

Alternative splicing operates by exon swapping and alternative 3' and 5' splice sites (e.g. in alternative forms of immunoglobulin). Regulation of alternative splicing is poorly understood. It is thought to involve transcription factors recognising specific RNA sequence elements, to suppress or express an exon.

16.1.5 Editing
Editing involves the changing of a nucleotide sequence of the mRNA molecule. This alters the coding of the mRNA molecule and thus encodes a different peptide from the same original gene. Examples include apoB100 and apoB48, important in lipid transport, which are formed from the same gene which may be edited in the small intestine to produce large and small proteins with different functions.

16.2 TRANSLATION
Translation is the process whereby a sequence of nucleotides on mRNA is converted into an amino acid sequence on a growing polypeptide chain.

mRNA is read in a 5' to 3' direction by ribosomes, which synthesise the corresponding protein from amino acids in the N to C-terminal direction. The amino acids are bound to tRNAs in aminoacyl-tRNA molecules, each of which bears a triplet of bases (anti-codon). The ribosome reads each triplet of the mRNA and an aminoacyl-tRNA with complimentary sequence binds to the transcript via hydrogen bonds. Peptides bonds are subsequently formed between the incoming amino acids and the growing end of the polypeptide chain.

Translation takes place in three stages:
- Initiation – formation of mRNA-ribosome complex, and the binding of the first codon (AUG) to the first aminoacyl-tRNA.
- Elongation – sequential reading of other codons and polypeptide growth by the addition of amino acids to the C-terminal end.
- Termination – stop codon needed, with no corresponding tRNA, so protein synthesis finishes and complete polypeptide can be released from the ribosome.

16.2.1 Aminoacyl-tRNAs
tRNA acts as a molecular adapter, with each tRNA having a cloverleaf structure stabilised by H-bonding. The anti-codon is in a highly accessible position.

Each tRNA carries a single amino acid at its 3' end, but due to the degenerate code several codons (and thus tRNAs) carry the same amino acid.

tRNA synthesis is performed by aminoacyl-tRNA synthase, which is important for adapter function and creation of high energy:

$$Amino\ acid + ATP + tRNA \rightarrow Aminoacyl\text{-}tRNA + AMP + PP_i$$

16.2.2 Ribosomes
Ribosomes are large ribonucleoprotein complexes on which proteins are synthesised. Their structure is conserved throughout evolution. In eukaryotes, ribosomes consist of 50 proteins and rRNAs (28S, 18S, 5.8S) which form into a large (50S) and small (30S) subunit.

Each ribosome has two sites for tRNA binding – an A site for aminoacyl-tRNA and a P site for peptidyl-tRNA linked to the growing peptide strand. Usually, ribosomes work in unison on an mRNA forming a 'polysome'.

16.2.3 The process of translation
1. Initiation
   - Small ribosomal subunit recognises and binds to mRNA complex with large subunit joining shortly afterwards.
   - The ribosome scans from the mRNA cap to the first AUG initiation codon.
   - Methionine tRNA is placed in the P site of the ribosome by initiation factors, which catalyse the formation of the initiation sequence on the small subunit. This requires energy from GTP hydrolysis. Together with the large subunit, this forms the 70S initiation complex.

2. Elongation
   - This involves three repeating steps:
     1. Aminoacyl-tRNA binds tightly to the A site of the ribosome, and base pairs with the mRNA. This requires ATP hydrolysis and elongation factors
     2. Formation of peptide bond between the incoming amino acid and the growing polypeptide chain at the P site, catalysed by peptidyl transferase (enzyme present in the large subunit).

161

3. Free tRNA leaves the P site, with the new peptidyl-tRNA in the A site being moved to the P site and ribosome shifting down in the 5' to 3' direction. Thus, the next codon to be read is over the A site:

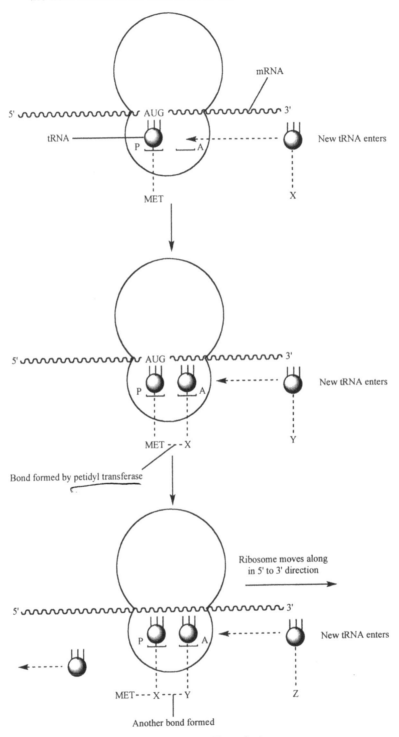

Figure 16.6 - Translation

3. Termination
    - Occurs when the stop codon (UAG, UAA or UGA) is reached since there is no complimentary tRNA.
    - Instead, one of two release factors bind, activating peptidyl transferase to cleave the bond between the polypeptide and tRNA at the P site.
    - Once cleavage has occurred, the polypeptide, tRNA and mRNA leave the ribosome, which dissociates into 30s and 50S subunits, ready to initiate translation again.

CHAPTER 17

Genome Organisation and Molecular Genetic Techniques

17.1 ORGANISATION OF THE GENOME

Genes are defined as the DNA information coding for an RNA transcript, plus the DNA motifs and epigenetic factors, which direct its transcription. The genome consists of a variety of different types of sequence:

Single copy sequences
- Most genes come as single copies and are dispersed throughout the genome. However, some genes with related structure and function (e.g. globin genes for haemoglobin) are found in clusters.

Multi-copy genes
- Some genes are present in multiple copies e.g. those that make rRNA and histone proteins.
- Tend to be genes that code for proteins required in large amounts – rRNA accounts for 80-90% of total RNA, and therefore genes for 28S, 18S and 5.8S rRNAs occur in huge tandem repeat sequences.

Non-coding sequences
- Many highly repeating non-coding sequences are present in the genome, such as simple sequence repeats (SSRs), retroelements (from viruses), short interspersed elements (SINEs) and segmental duplications.
- Large amount of the genome is non-coding, with only 1.5% being directly useful.

17.2 CHARACTERISATION OF GENES AT A MOLECULAR LEVEL

17.2.1 Cloning a DNA sequence

Cloning is the production of a large (and pure) amount of a certain stretch of DNA such that it may be used for other purposes.

17.2.1.1 Plasmid-based cloning

E. coli contain pieces of circular DNA, in addition to their normal genetic material, of around 3000 to 30000 base pairs. These are known as plasmids, and contain a single replication origin and thus replicate bi-directionally. These plasmids are not essential for life, with many being parasitic, but can carry useful genes such as those for antibiotic resistance.

E. coli plasmids can act as vehicles for foreign DNA, being implanted into cells and then replicated and reproduced many times as the bacteria replicate. The process of addition of a plasmid to a bacterium requires three steps:
1. Cutting, manipulating, isolating and joining the DNA.
2. Introduction of DNA into E. coli.
3. Purification of DNA from the E. coli population.

1. Cutting
- Done by one of 3500 restriction enzymes, which recognise a huge number of short sequence motifs, much like transcription factors.
- Found in virtually all bacteria, where they act as endonucleases in protection against viruses (methylation prevents spontaneous excision in vivo) – in culture conditions they can also acts as endonucleases, as long as Mg^{2+} is present in the medium.
- Cleavage by restriction enzymes occurs between restriction sites (4-6 base pairs long), producing restriction fragments that may be isolated. There are three types of ends produced from cutting:

5' overhangs e.g. EcoR1	5' GAATTC 3'	5' GA AATC 3'
	3' CTTAAG 5'	3' CTTAA G 5'
Blunt ends e.g. Fsp1	5' GAATTC 3'	5' GAA TTC 3'
	3' CTTAAG 5'	3' CTT AAG 5'
3' overhangs e.g. Kpn1	5' GAATTC 3'	5' GAAT TC 3'
	3' CTTAAG 5'	3' CT TAAG 5'

- Joining at 'sticky ends' to a plasmid can be done using DNA ligase as long as the ends of the sequences are compatible. This is done in a test tube using purified enzyme.
- Any blunt end can be ligated to any other blunt end, but incompatible overhangs cannot. Compatible ends of overhangs are adhesive since they form stable base pairs before ligation.

2. Uptake
- E. coli can be induced to take up the plasmid. Cells become competent to take up DNA from the environment by treatment with divalent cations (e.g. Ca^{2+}) and a brief heat shock of 42°C.
- Uptake of plasmids into cells can lead to stable maintenance of the new DNA in a process called transformation.

3. Purification
- E. coli plasmids are made to produce efficient cloning vectors e.g. through addition of antibiotic resistance.
- This can be used as a selective marker for cells containing the plasmid – addition of antibiotic to the medium kills cells which do not contain the plasmid.
- Purification of the plasmid from the cells is easy due to its small size relative to the rest of the genome:
  - Lyse cells with SDS and denature chromosomal DNA with alkali.
  - Neutralise lysate – intermolecular 're-naturation' causes chromosomes to precipitate out.
  - Remove cellular proteins by organic extraction and precipitate pure plasmid with salt and ethanol.

17.2.1.2 PCR-based cloning
The most important molecular biology technique is the polymerase chain reaction (PCR), which allows amplification of a specific sequence. This only requires knowledge of the nucleotide sequence of two primer regions.

PCR uses thermostable DNA polymerases from thermophilic hot spring bacteria, which are active at 72°C and can still operate at 95°C. PCR requires:
1. A template DNA strand
2. A pair of DNA primers
3. Four dNTPs
4. A thermostable polymerase

These ingredients are added together to a thermocycler – equipment that can accurately control the cycling between various temperatures and co-ordinate the timing of the reactions.

1. Preparation
   - Template DNA is melted by heating to 94°C, which denatures the DNA strand:

2. Primer binding
   - Reaction is cooled to a point at which the primers can base pair to complimentary sequences on the DNA template.
   - Normally around 45 to 55°C.

3. Strand synthesis
   - Reaction is raised to the optimum temperature for DNA polymerase to synthesise DNA – this is normally 72°C.
   - Elongation extends from both primers:

4. Strand separation
   - Reaction temperature is raised to 94°C again to melt all the DNA duplexes, thus doubling the number of template strands:

5. Repeat
   - Reaction is reduced to around 50°C again to allow primers to join all four template strands, and then the temperature is increased (as per step 3) to allow further synthesis to occur.
   - This is repeated 25 to 30 times to amplify the number of strands – there is an exponential increase, such that one chain can yield 1.1×10^9 copies in just 30 cycles.

PCR is cheap, quick and simple compared to cloning-based techniques. It can be used with the incorporation of dyes into sample sequences, allowing automated sequencing, quantitative analysis and diagnosis. In addition, it can be applied to archaeological and forensic study and amplification of long chain sequences. Importantly, PCR does not require exact knowledge of the template strand sequence and even the primers to do not have to be precise complimentary strands to operate effectively.

17.2.2 Electrophoresis

DNA molecules can be separated according to size with gel electrophoresis. The gel consists of a random 3D polymer meshwork suspended in an aqueous, electrically conductive buffer. When electrical current is passed through the gel, DNA pieces move through it, with the larger molecules being impeded more by the meshwork than the smaller ones – thus it acts like a 'molecular sieve'. The relative charge of the DNA fragments also affects their ability to traverse the gel.

Two types of gel are used – agarose (which has a low resolution) and polyacrylamide (with higher resolution). After the gel has been run, the DNA bands can be stained with UV-fluorescent substances. Marker DNA with a known molecular weight can be used as a reference.

17.2.3 Southern Blotting

After gel electrophoresis has been performed, there is often a need to detect one or more sequences. This is done by Southern blotting:

1. After electrophoresis, gel is soaked in alkali to denature the DNA to single strands, and is then neutralised.
2. Gel is placed in contact with a nitrocellulose or nylon membrane filter sheet, arranged so buffer flows through the gel carrying the DNA onto the membrane. This transfers the band pattern to the membrane, which can be peeled off and backed to fix the DNA.
3. Fixed DNA is incubated with a radiolabelled probe that binds to complimentary sequences – visualisation is carried out by washing away the probe and then placing filter membrane against X-ray film. This allows autoradiography to occur, such that the presence of tagged sequences can be confirmed.

Northern blotting is a similar process, only it is carried out with RNA molecules.

17.2.4 Probes

Probes are derived from cloned genes, and are used to investigate the structure and behaviour of the original gene in its genomic location. They are created by PCR in the presence of labelled dATP, such that every adenosine incorporated into the strand shows up as fluorescence. This can also be done with short oligonucleotide sequences, but the signal produced is not as bright.

17.2.5 DNA sequencing

DNA sequencing can reveal an entire DNA sequence of a gene or genes. It is based upon three core experimental approaches:

- Initiation of in vitro DNA synthesis with primer from a fixed point.
- Test tube synthesis of DNA with modified nucleotide.
- High resolution gel electrophoresis to detect different length nucleotides.

1. Cloning
   - Cloning of strand of DNA initiated and performed using E. coli and primer.

2. Heat
   - Cloned strands are separated by heating and alkali, and the radiolabelled sequencing primer is allowed to base pair.

3. Synthesis
   - DNA polymerase, four normal dNTPs and a small amount of dideoxynucleotide triphosphate (ddNTP) are added, and synthesis is allowed to occur.

168

- ddNTPs have no 3' OH, so when they are incorporated into the growing chain they stop synthesis.
- A mixture of labelled (via the primer) strands of various lengths are thus created, with termination occurring at every possible position for each nucleotide (depending on which ddNTP has been added – i.e. if ddATP then termination will occur only at adenosine residues so strand fragments with termination at each adenosine in the nucleotide sequence will occur).

4. Gel electrophoresis
   - Separation of each fragment using a high resolution electrophoresis, thus demonstrating the position of each of the specific nucleotides.

5. Repeat
   - Repeat process, using ddNTP for the other three nucleotides in turn.

Sequencing can now be done with each nucleotide represented by a different colour. Thus, computers can run automated scans to sequence a sample extremely quickly.

CHAPTER 18

Concepts in Medical Genetics and Chromosome Diseases

18.1 GENERAL CONCEPTS OF MEDICAL GENETICS

In the developed world, as infectious diseases recede, genetic disorders are becoming more important contributors to morbidity and mortality, especially in children. This is because many prevalent diseases such as diabetes, hypertension and arthritis have a genetic basis.

There is a balance between genetic and environmental interaction, such as with skin cancer, in which genetics can predispose to the disease but exposure to the sun is required for pathogenesis.

18.1.1 Fundamentals of Mendelian Genetics

Character – the characteristic or feature that a certain gene codes for e.g. eye colour.

Gene – physical unit of heredity, which codes for a specific RNA and is thus necessary for protein production molecularly, and encodes for a certain characteristic or phenotype macroscopically.

Allele – one, two or more alternative forms of the same gene, located at the corresponding locus on homologous chromosomes.

Genotype – the genetic constitution of an individual organism, as represented by the allele characteristic for an individual (the combination of alleles for a certain gene e.g. AA vs Aa).

Phenotype – characteristic or biochemical feature resulting from the interaction of its genotype with its environment.

Dominant trait – traits which are expressed (i.e. phenotype present) when an individual is heterozygous.

Recessive trait – traits only expressed in individuals that are homozygous for the certain allele, and thus people who are heterozygous typically possess normal phenotype and are only carriers.

18.1.2 Other Definitions

Consanguineous – describes the closeness of relationship between two individuals. Two people are consanguineous if they share parents or grandparents.

Penetrance – describes the movement of a genetic disease through a pedigree (generation to generation within a family). If a parent has a normal phenotype, but their child is affected by a disease it is known as incomplete penetrance. This only applies to autosomal dominant diseases, and is due to tandem repeat accumulation e.g. Huntington's Disease.

Expression – dominant diseases affect different tissues and different individuals to a variable extent within a generation. This is called variable expression or expressivity.

Heteroplasmy – mixture of mutant and normal cells or organelles within a cell, resulting in different tissues being affected in different ways e.g. brain > bone in mitochondrial diseases such as MELAS and MERRF.

18.2 CHROMOSOMES

18.2.1 General

Chromosomes are the highest form of DNA coiling, and in each species there is a set number and size of chromosome complement (karyotype). Chromosome structure can be thought of as hierarchical, much like the structure of proteins, with various levels of motif formation and packaging.

Metaphase chromosomes can be grouped according to the position of their centromere:
- Metacentric – centromere at the centre e.g. chromosome 3.
- Submetacentric – centromere away from the centre e.g. chromosome 17 and 18.
- Acrocentric – centromere at the end of the chromosome, often with a stalk and satellite region e.g. chromosome 21 and 22.

There are various regions within a chromosome's structure which can be identified by staining and other techniques, which are important for function in vivo. These include:
- P-arm – 'petite' short arm of the chromosome.
- Q-arm – larger arm of the chromosome.
- Centromere – holds two sister chromatids together during meiosis and mitosis and often contains satellite short repeating DNA sequences.
- GC-rich light regions.
- AT-rich dark regions.
- Banding – different regions within the chromosome and the different levels of activity of the genes within them according to density of packaging. Demonstrated using Giemsa staining techniques (trypsin followed by stain), and are numbered to allow definition of a particular region e.g. p12 = band 12 on p-arm of a chromosome.
- Telomeres – regions at the ends of chromosomes consisting of protein-DNA complexes that shield the chromosome from end degradation and end-to-end fusion with other chromosomes.

18.2.2 Normal complement and sex determination
The human karyotype consists of 46 (23 pairs) of chromosomes. There are 22 homologous pairs of autosomes that are numbered according to size – with 1 the largest – and one pair of sex chromosomes (X and Y).

The X-chromosome is large, containing 6% of the total DNA in a cell. There are over 300 genes on an X-chromosome, and almost 250 diseases are known to be X-linked. The Y-chromosome is much smaller, with only 26 functional genes and less than 20 known Y-linked diseases. Importantly, the Y-chromosome contains the sex-determining Y region (SRY), which encodes transcription factors for the development of male internal and external genitalia.

The existence of a single Y-chromosome stimulates the formation of a male foetus, and thus even 49,XXXXY individuals (if this karyotype were compatible with life) would be male.

18.3 CHROMOSOME DISORDERS
Chromosome abnormalities are frequent and often problematic. They account for 50% of early miscarriages, 5% of still births and 0.5% of abnormalities at live birth. Chromosomal disorders can occur by three mechanisms
- Misrepair or broken chromosomes.
- Improper recombination.
- Malsegregation during mitosis or meiosis.

Any one of these three factors can lead to chromosome-associated problems, which can themselves be divided into two groups:
- Structural abnormalities
- Numerical abnormalities

The expression of chromosomal disorder phenotypes is due to a gene dosage effect. In many cases,

172

a chromosomal malfunction results in a silent mutation – i.e. one with no discernible phenotype. However, in order for normal development to take place, innumerable tightly controlled interactions between gene products must occur and, if a gene is under or over-expressed, this process may be disrupted leading to disease.

18.3.1 Numerical Chromosome Disorders
Ploidy describes the number of chromosomes that a person has:
- Euploidy – refers to any exact multiple of n, where n is the number of chromosomes in a haploid cell (23 in humans).
- Diploidy – number of chromosomes in a normal somatic cell (2n).
- Polyploidy – increased number of haploid sets beyond dipolidy e.g. triploidy where there are three sets, and thus 69 chromosomes in total.
- Aneuploidy – any number of chromosomes that is not euploid and normal, resulting from a lack (monosomy) or gain (trisomy) of a single chromosome.

18.3.1.1 Aneuploidy
Aneuploidy is thought to arise due to non-dysjunction, where a pair of bivalent chromosomes fails to separate either during meiosis or mitosis. This results in the formation of one otherwise diploid cell with three copies of a particular chromosome, and one daughter cell with only one copy of that chromosome.

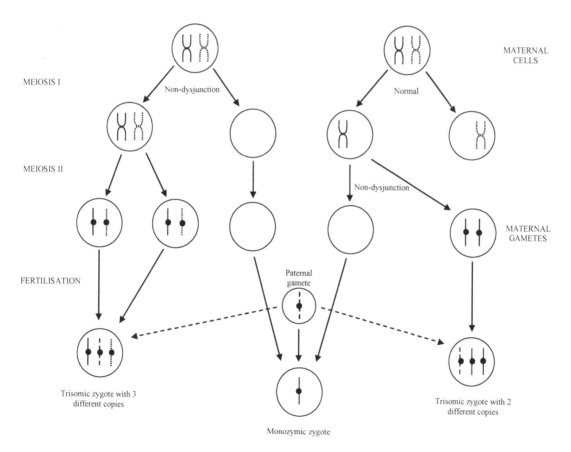

Figure 18.1 – Non-dysjunction and aneuploidy

The timing of non-dysjunction is very important. If it occurs during meiosis I and II of gametogenesis, it results in a constitutional condition that is present in all body cells. If, however, it occurs during mitosis in early embryonic growth a mosaic of normal and aneuploid cells results. This means that a constitutively lethal condition may become compatible with life since only some somatic cells are affected.

Trisomies

Down's Syndrome
The most common example of trisomy (and thus aneuploidy) is Down's syndrome, caused by trisomy 21. This affects 1 in 800 live births, with an increased risk with increase in maternal age. 90% of cases are due to an additional chromosome 21 from the mother due to meiotic non-dysjunction in meiosis I. The other 10% are due to an unbalanced translocation of the long arm of chromosome 21 with chromosomes 13, 14 or 15 and mosaicism (non-dysjunction during mitosis in early embryo development). This occurs randomly in 60% of cases, but can be inherited making it important to family members, since they may be carriers.

Symptoms
- Growth and mental retardation.
- Significant congenital heart defects e.g. atrioventricular canal defects.
- Somatic features – head, face, single palmar crease, epicanthal folds.
- Features of Alzheimer's disease past 35 years.
- Decreased life expectancy (<60 years).

Mechanism
- Additional genetic material results in the over-expression of certain gene products from the 1500 genes on chromosome 21.
- Superoxide dismutase is an enzyme which breaks down free radicals to O_2 and H_2O_2. In the Down's foetal brain tissue, high SOD levels mean there is an abundance of H_2O_2 which is able to cause free radical damage to lipids. This impairs the function and structure of cerebral cortex neurone membranes leading to premature cortical ageing in Down's syndrome.
- Amyloid precursor protein is over-expressed, which is likely to be associated with the Alzheimer's symptoms.
- α-A-crystallin build up leads to cataract development.
- Oncogene ETS-2 leads to increased prevalence of leukaemia.

Others
Very few trisomies survive to term, but other life-compatible defects include trisomy 13 (Patau's syndrome) and 18 (Edward's syndrome). These diseases are characterised by severe mental retardation, cardiac abnormalities and early death. These trisomies are only possible as all three chromosomes contain very few genes – trisomies of chromosomes in which there are more functional genes result in spontaneous abortion.

Monosomies
Monosomies in autosomes are invariably lethal. On every chromosome, there are a number of genes where halving the gene product in incompatible with development. Often, halving a single gene product is not sufficient to cause death, but a combination of effects results in disruption of normal embryonic development.

174

Sex chromosome abnormalities

Abnormalities in the sex chromosomes are much less severe than similar autosomal conditions. This is because the Y-chromosome contains very few gene products, and random X-chromosome inactivation controls the level of X-chromosome gene product independent of the number of chromosomes present. Thus, 45,XO for example with no X inactivation shows near normal levels of gene product.

Abnormality	Sex	Features
47,XYY	Male	- 1 in 1000 live male births. - Normal sexual development and fertile. - Tall stature, mild retardation and extreme aggressive nature. - Due to paternal meiotic non-dysjunction.
47,XXY – Klinefelter's	Male	- 1 in 1000 male live births. - Accounts for 10% of male infertility. - Small testes, breast enlargement, azoospermia after puberty, long limbs and mental retardation.
47,XXX	Female	- Fertile and normal, but a reduced IQ.
45,XO – Turner's	Female	- 1 in 5000 live female births, but >99% spontaneously abort - Gonadal dysgenesis, infertility, sexual immaturity, amenorrhoea and short stature. - May be due to structural defects too, and many patients are mosaics of 46,XX and 45,XO. - Develops even though X-inactivation occurs in normal females because certain genes require both chromosomes for a sufficient gene dosage effect e.g. those for ovarian development, female puberty. These are homologous with those present on the Y-chromosome.

18.3.1.2 Polyploidy

1-3% of all recognised human pregnancies are triploid, with three full sets of chromosomes. They may be caused by failure of gametes to undergo meiosis. In humans, babies rarely survive to term (in contrast to plants, where triploidy actually results in more rigorous and successful strains). Any individual that does survive to term is sterile. This is because three sets of chromosomes are unable to pair up and segregate properly in meiosis.

In humans, the origin of the additional genetic material affects the way that the polyploidy presents. It is thought this relies on epigenetic imprinting:
- Paternal origin – placental swelling to support the baby and 'discard' the mother.
- Maternal origin – small placenta, with foetus less likely to survive in order to protect the mother.

When a zygote is formed that contains a diploid chromosome set, but only from one parent (i.e. a clone) the result is a hydratidiform mole (when of paternal origin) or an ovarian teratoma (when of maternal origin). These are benign tumours of differentiated and partially differentiated tissues and can be seen in the womb as discordant collections of hair, teeth, neurones and other structures.

18.3.2 Structural Chromosome Disorders
Structural chromosome problems may affect only a small region of a particular chromosome, or involve one or more chromosomes. They can results from misrepair of chromosome breaks or malfunction of the recombination system.

There are various different types of structural chromosome disorders:
- Single chromosome
  - Deletion
  - Duplication
  - Pericentric inversion (with centromere)
  - Paracentric inversion (without centromere)
  - Ring chromosome formation
  - Isochromosome formation
- Two or more chromosomes
  - Insertion from one to another.
  - Translocation or exchange of material – reciprocal or Robertsonian translocations.

Clinically, it is much more important to classify chromosome disorders according to their effects:
- Balanced abnormalities – no net loss or gain of chromosomal material.
- Unbalanced abnormalities – change in the amount of chromosome material resulting in a net gene dose effect.

18.3.2.1 Balanced abnormalities
In balanced abnormalities, the normal diploid number of genes is present, so an individual is phenotypically normal unless an important functional gene is directly affected. However, passing on of a balanced rearrangement may cause an unbalanced abnormality in offspring e.g. extra chromosome 21 on the short arm of chromosome 14 via Robertsonian translocation leading to trisomy 21 in offspring.

Reciprocal translocation
Reciprocal translocation involves the breakage of two chromosomes and the exchange of genetic material forming two new derivative chromosomes, with no net loss or gain of genetic material. Importantly, this only happens to one of a pair of homologous chromosomes, leading to a karyotype with one translocation chromosome and one normal chromosome.

At meiosis, a cross-shaped structure is thus formed and in gametogenesis the homologous chromosomes can separate in a number of ways:
- Normal gamete formation.
- Balanced translocation passed on to gamete so no problem.
- One normal and one translocation chromosome in a gamete, leading to alteration in amount of a certain piece of genetic material. This leads to an unbalanced abnormality in the foetus when the gamete is fertilised and symptoms of chromosomal disorders (e.g. Down's) can occur. However, sperm with unbalanced translocations are often destroyed in the uterus before fertilisation can occur.

An example of reciprocal translocation is that between chromosome 9 and 22 (creating the Philadelphia chromosome), which results in chronic myeloid leukaemia.

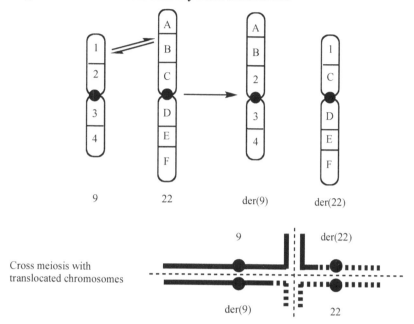

Figure 18.2 – Reciprocal translocation and meiosis with translocated chromosomes

Robertsonian translocation
Robertsonian translocation describes the breakage of the short arms of two chromosomes, with the fusion of the long arms. This is also known as centric fusion.

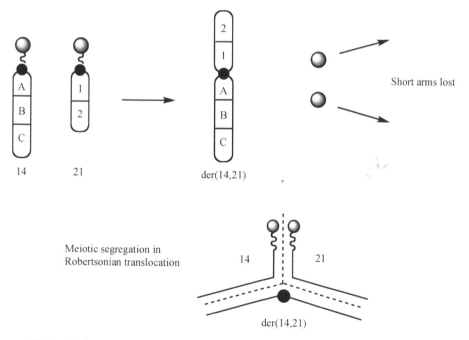

Figure 18.3 – Robertsonian translocation and meiosis in translocated chromosomes

Robertsonian translocation involves D and G group chromosomes (13, 14, 15, 21 and 22) since they are acrocentric, meaning they tend to cluster during meiosis, allowing breakage and fusion (with resultant loss of the short arms) to occur. Molecularly, this type of translocation is unbalanced since the short arms are lost. However, since satellite DNA in acrocentric chromosomes encodes for redundant proteins, individuals with these translocations are phenotypically normal.

Again, this type of translocation may result in problems for offspring due to abnormal meiosis occurring and the formation of unbalanced gametes. This is a major mechanism for Down's syndrome pathogenesis without trisomy, since three copies of the long arm of chromosome 21 can be present when translocations between chromosome 14 and 21 occur.

Inversions
Inversions involve two break rearrangements, involving only a single chromosome in which the segment is reversed. This is a balanced abnormality, assuming the breakage point (and thus inversion segment) does not change any actual functional gene.

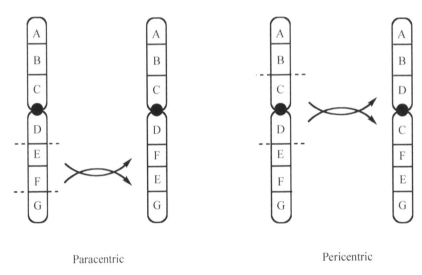

Paracentric   Pericentric

Figure 18.4 - Inversions

18.3.2.2 Unbalanced abnormalities
The consequences of unbalanced abnormalities are often severe and deleterious since the incorrect amount of genetic material is present, leading to a gene dosage effect and disease.

Isochromosomes
Isochromosomes occur when the centromere of a chromosome divides transversely instead of longitudinally, such that one arm of the chromosome is missing and the other arm is duplicated. The chromosomes formed have two arms with the same loci, but the sequences are reversed:

178

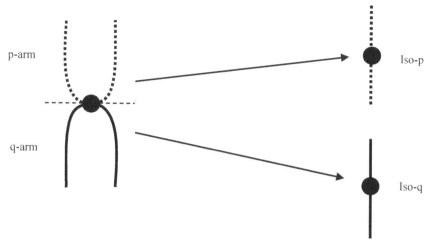

Figure 18.5 – Isochromosome formation

When this occurs in autosomes, it is often lethal. However, the most common form of the abnormality occurs in the X-chromosome, resulting in a phenotype similar to Turner's syndrome. This develops because of the under-expression of the genetic material present on the arm of the chromosome that is lost.

Deletions
Deletion causes part of a chromosome to be lost, resulting in under-expression of certain genes. The severity of the disease depends on the nature and extent of genetic loss, with >2% genome loss resulting in death of the foetus due to absence of functionally important proteins. Microdeletions usually involve a few genes at closely related loci and produce a variety of cell characterised syndromes.

CATCH 22 syndrome
- Associated with deletion of chromosome 22q11.2.
- Present with <u>c</u>ardiac defects, <u>a</u>bnormal facies, <u>t</u>hymic hypoplasia, <u>c</u>left palate and <u>h</u>ypoc-alcaemia.
- In addition, it includes DiGeorge and craniofacial syndromes.
- Incidence of 1 in 5000, representing 5% of congenital heart defects.
- Pathogenesis because chromosome 22 required for branchial arch development.
- Diagnosis and detection by FISH.

Duchenne muscular dystrophy
- X-linked disease with Xp21.2 deletion.
- Genetic defect demonstrated by studies into rare girls with Duchenne muscular dystrophy and cloning analysis.

Cri du chat
- Chromosome 5 deletion.

Prader-Willi syndrome
- Microdeletion in chromosome 15q11-q13.
- Occurs in 1 in 10000 live births.

- Present with moderate retardation, hypotonia, poor feeding followed by obesity after 2 years, small genitalia, hands and feet.
- Deletion always inherited from the child's father.

Angelman syndrome
- Same deletion as Prader-Willi syndrome, but maternally inherited.
- Present with severe mental retardation, seizures, jerky gait, inappropriate laughter and large tongue.
- Comparison with Prader-Willi syndrome illustrates the idea of genomic imprinting via methylation, which preferentially activates or inactivates certain genes. Thus, combination of microdeletion in paternal allele, plus maternal methylation (inactivates the genes) leads to effectively no function copy of that region of chromosome 15, and subsequently Prader-Willi syndrome.

Duplications
Duplications are much more common than deletions, and less harmful since there is no net genetic loss. There are two types – direct (tandem) and inverted (mirror) duplications:

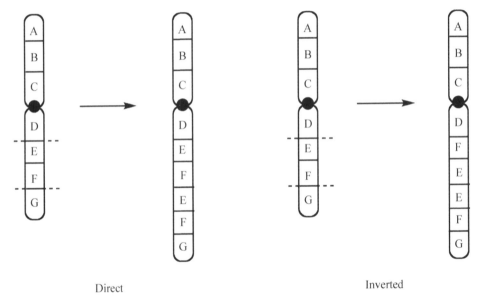

Direct   Inverted

Figure 18.6 - Duplications

Fragile chromosome disorders
Fragile chromosome disorders are those in which chromosome damage accumulates throughout the patient's life.

An important example is Fragile X Syndrome. This affects 1 in 1250 males, and 1 in 2000 females, and is associated with damage at Xq27.3. The disease presents with mental retardation, facial abnormalities and large testes in males. It is another example of genetic imprinting, as it only occurs in women if it is maternally inherited.

Other fragile chromosome diseases include Bloom's syndrome, Fanconi's anaemia and Xeroderma Pigmentosa.

180

18.3.3 Chromosome abnormalities, cancer and spontaneous abortions

Various cancers are associated with abnormalities in chromosomes, such as the Philadelphia chromosome in chronic myeloid leukaemia and Burkitt's lymphoma, where reciprocal translocation leads to proto-oncogene activation. In addition, cells which become cancerous can transform into aneuploid cells.

Major clinical consequences can occur with chromosome abnormalities, even before birth. Over 50% of spontaneous abortions are due to chromosome problems, and approximately 25% of all conceptions are affected by major chromosome abnormalities.

The most common causes of spontaneous abortion are trisomy 16 and 45,XO. However, trisomy 13, 18 and 21, 47,XXX, 47,XXY and 47,XYY can also result in abortion along with triploidy and tetraploidy.

CHAPTER 19

Genetics of Disease

19.1 SINGLE GENE DISORDERS

Single gene disorders are those which are due to a mutation in one or both of a pair of autosomal genes, or due to a mutation in an X or Y chromosome gene. Since the pathogenesis of these diseases involves only a single gene, they follow Mendelian inheritance patterns.

19.1.1 Autosomal Dominant Disorders

A single gene disease is autosomal dominant if heterozygotes express the disease phenotype.

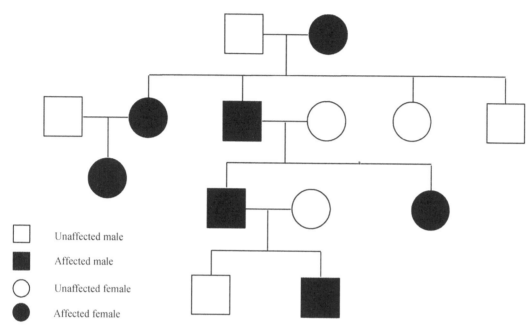

□ Unaffected male

■ Affected male

○ Unaffected female

● Affected female

Figure 19.1 – Autosomal dominant inheritance

Features
- Males and females affected equally.
- Affected individuals in each generation, and males can pass to males or females and vice versa.
- Unaffected individuals do not transmit the disease – no carrier state.

Examples
- Osteogenesis imperfecta – 1 in 10,000.
- Huntington's disease – 5 in 10,000.
- Familial hypercholesterolaemia – 20 in 10,000.
- Over 4500 autosomal dominant diseases known.

Segregation
- Mendelian experiments demonstrate that autosomal dominant characteristics show distinct units of inheritance i.e. single gamete from mother, single gamete from father with traits not continuous spectrum but distinct.

Penetrance
- Describes the effect of the mutation on the phenotype of an individual.

- Non-penetrance – individual has the mutant gene, but does not express the phenotype. They can, however, pass the mutation to the next generation.
- Variable penetrance – disease is age-dependent (e.g. Huntington's) or increases through generations.
- Total penetrance – every individual with the mutation presents with the disease or phenotype.

Expressivity
- Variation in expression occurs with autosomal dominant disease.
- Expressivity describes the variation in time of onset and severity of the disease.

Risk to offspring
- Homozygous normal, heterozygous affected → 50% of offspring affected.
- Homozygous normal, homozygous affected → 100% affected.
- Both homozygous affected → all offspring affected, and potential spontaneous abortion.

19.1.2 Autosomal Recessive Disorders
AR diseases are characterised by the presence of carriers, with the affected gene being present on an autosomal chromosome.

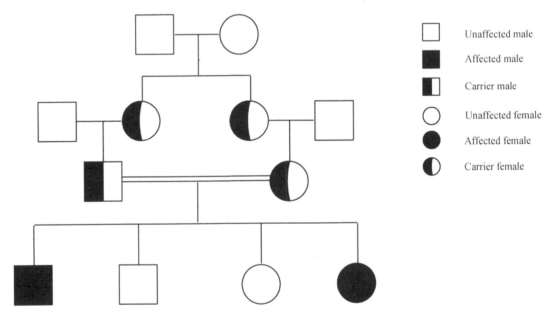

Figure 19.2 – Autosomal recessive inheritance

Features
- Affected individuals can have unaffected parents.
- 25% risk to siblings if an individual is found to be affected.
- Equal number of males and females affected.
- Often due to consanguinity – intra-family mating increases the chance of presenting with the disease.
- Often cause enzyme defects.

184

- 50% loss of function in heterozygotes still allows normal function, so only homozygotes are affected.
- Heterozygotes can be carriers of the allele, and pass on the disease to offspring.

Examples
- Phenylketonuria – 1.2 in 10,000.
- Tay-Sachs disease – 0.04 in 10,000.
- Cystic fibrosis – 5 in 10,000 (but 1 in 22 are carriers).
- Sickle cell anaemia – 1 in 10,000.
- Thalassemia – 0.5 in 10,000.
- In total there are believed to be over 1700 autosomal recessive disorders.

19.1.3 X-linked Disorders
X-linked diseases are those in which the affected gene is present on the X-chromosome, leading to an increased prevalence in males.

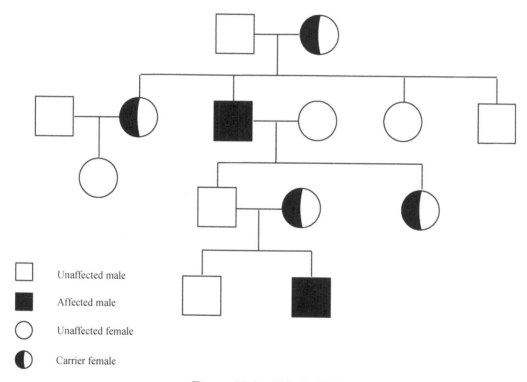

Figure 19.3 – X-linked inheritance

Features
- Each daughter must receive the paternal X-chromosome, whilst each son must receive the paternal Y-chromosome meaning males can only get the disease from their mother.
- No male to male transmission.
- Carrier mother with a normal father → 50% of daughters are carriers whilst 50% of sons are affected.
- In rare circumstances, females can be homozygous, or have Turner's syndrome (45,X0) and therefore express the disease phenotype.

185

Examples
- Duchenne muscular dystrophy – 3 in 10,000.
- Haemophilia A and B – 2 in 10,000.
- Fragile X mental retardation – 5 in 10,000.

19.1.4 Mitochondrial Inheritance
Features
- Mitochondrial genome and mitochondria are maternally inherited, meaning that affected mother passes on the disease.
- Phenotype depends upon the location, type of mutation and proportion, allowing hetero-plasmy (different levels of affected mitochondria in different cells) to develop.
- Affect mainly the CNS, heart, skeletal muscle, kidney and endocrine tissues.

Examples
- MERRF 0.1 in 10,000.
- LON 0.3 in 10,000.
- 59 diseases have been identified.

19.1.5 Polygenic Diseases
Polygenic, or multifactorial, traits are those controlled and affected by a number of genes, and their interactions with the environment.

Polygenic diseases can be investigated using twin studies to identify the relative contribution of environment and genes (the heritability) to a phenotype. This involves comparison of monozygotic (i.e. same genes and same environment) and dizygotic (i.e. same environment only) twins.

19.2 GENES IN POPULATIONS

19.2.1 Allele Frequency
The frequency of an allele can vary greatly, and it can thus directly affect the prevalence of a given disease. Allele frequency is determined by the following characteristics in the phenotype for which it encodes:
- Birth incidence
- Age of onset
- Longevity

Birth incidence can vary widely between ethnic groups (e.g. CF 1 in 2,000 in Western populations, but 1 in 10,000 in the Far East). This is thought to be due to:
- Allele frequency
- Mode of inheritance
- Penetrance
- Breeding patterns
- Fitness (the effect of the mutation, and how well it is passed on)
- New mutation rate

19.2.2 Hardy-Weinberg Equilibrium
The Hardy-Weinberg equilibrium is used to describe allele variation within populations. It predicts that in a large population in which there is no gene flow (closed system), random mating, no mutation

and no selection, the frequency of alleles (and thus of homo and heterozygotes) is stable and predictable over generations.

The Hardy-Weinberg equilibrium can be expressed in equation form, with normal allele A having a frequency p, and disease allele a having a frequency q:

$$p + q = 1$$

Frequencies of individuals:

$$AA = p^2$$
$$Aa = 2pq$$
$$Aa = q^2$$

And therefore $p^2 + 2pq + q^2 = 1$

It can be shown mathematically that these frequencies do not change over time. However, the ideal conditions on which the equilibrium relies are rarely met and thus deviation leads to variation in allele frequencies.

19.2.2.1 Small population size
Several rare autosomal recessive disorders show a higher incidence in certain populations and communities, which are isolated geographically and reproductively. An example of this is the Ashkenazi Jew population, in which there is a high prevalence of Tay-Sachs disease, characterised by sphingolipidosis leading to mental and motor retardation with blindness.

There are a number of theories for how this increased incidence may occur. The 'founder effect' has been proposed, in which certain genetic diseases are more common in particular populations since all individuals are descended from the same small number of ancestors. If one or more of these ancestors possessed a disease allele, it would appear with a relatively increased frequency.

Similarly, genetic drift has been suggested. If one allele fails to pass to the next generation, it disappears from the population leaving only a single allele. This causes random fluctuation in allele frequency, depending on which individuals have offspring. Thus, there can be significant loss or fixation of one particular allele if all the carriers of the same allele are unable or decide not to reproduce. Also, small populations may lead to non-random mating, with geographical, political and religious isolation leading to breeding within a small gene pool.

19.2.2.2 Non-random mating
Mating is seldom a random process. Associative mating occurs naturally, with members of a particular sub-group of a population more likely to reproduce due to shared ethnic, racial, religious or other characteristics. Also, mating may be based on intelligence, or congenital deafness, for example, leading to small increases in the frequency of affected individuals.

Consanguinity – marriage between blood relatives – leads to an increase in the frequency of affected homozygotes, although allele frequency stays the same. An historical example of this is haemophilia within the Russian monarchy.

19.2.2.3 Selection
Selection may take the form of positive or negative pressure, to increase or decrease allele frequency.

Negative selective pressure operates to reduce the frequency of disadvantageous alleles, with the biggest effects being in autosomal dominant disorders. For example, infertility occurs in cystic fibrosis (congenital lack of vas in males, cilia immotility in females) and some autosomal dominant diseases are associated with death before reproductive age or disability preventing reproduction.

Positive selection may favour the survival of an allele in the population, despite its differential or disease-causing effects. Late-onset diseases such as Huntington's experience no negative pressure, since the disease presents beyond reproductive age, and thus the allele frequency stays consistent. Moreover, disease-phenotype may afford some protection against environmental pressures e.g. sickle cell trait and malaria, CF and cholera, PKU and spontaneous abortion, Tay-Sachs and TB.

19.2.2.4 New alleles
New alleles may enter a gene pool by two mechanisms:
- Migration – the diffusion of alleles across a racial or geographical boundary has been demonstrated for diseases including thalassemia, leading to gradual changes in gene frequency from Asia to Europe.
- Mutation – new mutations maintain lethal genetic diseases in a population. Some genes show particularly high mutation rates, such as the DMD gene (1×10^4 mutations) due to the large size of the gene, providing a larger target for mutagenic agents.

19.2.2.5 Future considerations
Given our increasing understanding of genetic disease, and important factors in its prevalence, it is important to consider how we might alter allele frequency. Treatments for genetic disease might allow affected individuals to reproduce, or even facilitate homozygote mating. In the case of CF, for example, this would increase the incidence of the allele.

However, screening programs could have the reverse effect. Detection of Tay-Sachs carrier status amongst Ashkenazi Jews allows individuals to decide whether to have children or not. Similarly, prenatal diagnosis and the option to terminate would reduce the frequency of disease alleles in the population.

19.3 THE HUMAN GENOME, MAPPING AND DIAGNOSIS

19.3.1 DNA Polymorphisms
Polymorphisms in genetics describes the presence of two or more distinct phenotypes in a population due to the expression of different alleles of a given gene, such as human blood groups O, A, B, and AB. Polymorphisms within sequences of DNA can be used to distinguish two individuals, and are responsible for variation between members of a population.

19.3.1.1 Restriction Fragment Length Polymorphisms
Genetic markers can, in principle, be any polymorphic locus. However, genetic mapping depends heavily on DNA markers – these are loci at which the alleles vary in the population, and can be readily distinguished from one another by a variety of techniques.

Restriction fragment length polymorphisms (RFLPs) are the simplest set of markers. They rely on DNA sequence variation between chromosomes at defined Restriction Enzyme target sites, allowing for two alleles – one where the enzyme is able to cut the chromosome, and one where the enzyme can not cut. Once the DNA sample has been treated with enzyme, it undergoes electrophoresis and Southern blotting.

188

However, RFLPs provide only two alleles, making it less useful, and crosses between homozygous parents can not be told apart using this marker (important in identifying the father of a child).

19.3.1.2 Single Nucleotide Polymorphisms

Single nucleotide polymorphisms (SNPs) do not rely on variants occurring at restriction enzyme sites. They simply represent variation in bases at a set of defined sites. However, like RFLPs, there are a limited number of alleles at each site reducing the specificity of the test.

19.3.1.3 Micro and Mini-satellites

Micro and mini-satellite sequences are composed of tandemly repeating DNA segments. Thus, they represent a variable number of tandem repeats (VNTR) system, with the number of repeats varying from allele to allele.

Multiple different alleles are identifiable following amplification via PCR and electrophoresis. As such, this technique is used for genetic fingerprinting of criminals and in paternity testing.

19.3.2 Genetic Linkage

Linkage

Mendel's Law of Segregation states that alleles at one locus segregate into gametes independently of alleles at another locus. However, the closer two loci are together, the more likely they are to be passed on together (along with their phenotype). This is known as genetic linkage, and allows approximation of the distance between two genes, and thus their relative positions. This technique may be used in genetic mapping.

Diseases

Linkage can be used to identify the position of disease-causing genes, such that (via the distance between two genes), the risk estimate for developing a disease can be calculated. For example, if a father has familial hypercholesterolaemia plus another particular (and identifiable) phenotype, if his offspring has the same phenotype, one can predict the chance of the child also suffering from familial hypercholesterolaemia.

19.4 MUTATION AND HUMAN DISEASE

19.4.1 Single Base Changes

Single base substitution is a frequent cause of disease when base changes alter the amino acid sequence. Often, single base changes do not cause harm and thus merely represent polymorphisms within a population.

If a mutation does change the amino acid sequence in such as way as to have a negative effect, the resulting gene product is likely to show loss of function (e.g. inactive enzyme). In addition, mutation may also result in gain of function (e.g. achondroplasia), with the gene product showing lack of sensitivity to inhibition or inactivation.

Sickle cell anaemia
- Single base change from GAG to GTG leading to a glutamine to valine change in amino acid in the haemoglobin polypeptide sequence.
- Haemoglobin becomes less soluble in water since valine is non-polar, and thus at low partial pressures of oxygen, the polypeptide forms long polymers which may deform red cells leading to haemolysis and obstruction to small vessels.

-   Sickle cell changes do, however, lead to resistance to malaria.

β-thalassemia
-   Single base substitution leading to the insertion of a stop codon, and subsequently ineffective β-globin synthesis.
-   Can also be caused by a mutation in splice sites, leading to short and unstable β-globin.

19.4.2 Deletions and Frame Shifts
Small (e.g. CF) or large (e.g. DMD) sections of a gene may be deleted, leading to disease. If small deletions occur in anything other than multiples of 3, a frame shift occurs, meaning that the gene downstream of the mutation has the incorrect amino acid sequence and is functionless. In addition, a stop codon may be inserted, abbreviating the gene product. Milder phenotypes result from deletions in multiples of three.

19.4.3 Anticipation
Micro-satellite repeat regions are dynamic since they change, with an increase or decrease in the number of repeats, leading to alteration in the length of the repeat region. An expanding section can mean that, once the micro-satellite reaches threshold level from one generation to the next, the disease phenotype presents. Thus, a disease may get increasingly common or severe through generations. An example of this is Huntington's disease, in the male germ line.

19.4.4 Dominant vs. Recessive Disorders
Whether a disease is dominant or recessive is dependent on the phenotypic effect of a change in 50% of the gene product (whether that be complete loss, or alteration in function):
-   50% activity sufficient for normal function → recessive.
-   50% activity insufficient, or mutated product interferes with other genes (dominant negative effect) → dominant.

In general, dominant diseases tend to affect structural proteins rather than enzymes due to the above phenomenon. For example, osteogenesis imperfecta and Marfan's syndrome are both AD diseases of connective tissue proteins.

CHAPTER 20

Haemostasis

20.1 HAEMOSTASIS

Haemostasis is the process by which bleeding from an injured vessel is arrested or reduced. This involves a sequence of events:

1. Vascular spasm.
2. Platelet aggregation, activation and release of chemical mediators.
3. The blood coagulation cascade.
4. Localisation of the clot that has formed.
5. Removal of the clot, allowing for wound repair.

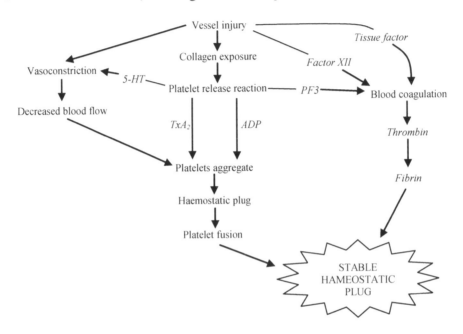

This has to be tightly regulated, with defects in the haemostatic system leading to bleeding disorders such as haemophilia, or aberrant coagulation leading to thrombosis.

20.2 VASCULAR SPASM AND THE BLOOD VESSEL ENDOTHELIUM

20.2.1 Vessel Constriction

Injury to the endothelium of a vessel leads to a local contractile response, with the smooth muscle causing the vessel to narrow. In addition, the upstream arterioles and small arteries constrict, limiting blood flow to the damaged areas. These processes are rapid and short-lived and are designed to limit bleeding, by preventing blood from flowing to the damaged area. The reduced blood flow also facilitates contact activation of platelets and coagulation factors.

After the initial trigger (i.e. trauma) has been removed, local factors such as serotonin, bradykinin and thromboxane A_2 from platelets maintain vasoconstriction.

20.2.2 Blood Vessel Endothelium

Under normal circumstances, the blood vessel endothelium helps to prevent coagulation from occurring. Surface heparan sulphate (a surface glycosaminoglycan related to the drug heparin) acts as a co-factor for antithrombin III (see below) and thus prevents platelet aggregation and coagulation cascade initiation.

However, the blood vessel endothelium also synthesises and stores many pro-thrombogenic molecules, which may be released on damage or activation, and thus accelerate clot formation:
- Tissue factor – released on damage to the endothelium, and activates the 'extrinsic' clotting pathway.
- Von Willebrand factor – glycoprotein synthesised in vascular endothelial cells and platelets, which enables binding of platelets to damaged vessels (binds to glycoprotein Ib receptors on the platelet surface).
- Plasminogen activator inhibitor 1 – PAI-1 which is secreted in response to angiotensin IV, providing a link between the renin-angiotensin system (used to regulate blood pressure) and clotting. Plasminogen activator is important in the breakdown of clots, and thus PAI-1 inhibits the removal of clots that are forming.
- Collagen – exposure of collagen on damage to blood vessels, leading to aggregation of platelets through binding to receptors on their surface.

Once clots have formed, the vascular endothelium also plays a role in limiting the extension of coagulation and its resolution to allowing healing to occur:
- Prostaglandin I_2 and nitric oxide – convert platelet agonist ADP to adenosine, which can inhibit platelet function.
- Tissue plasminogen activator – synthesised by the vascular endothelium and accelerates plasmin formation and clot removal.
- Thrombomodulin – receptor for thrombin, which, in combination with thrombin, activates the vitamin K-dependent anticoagulant, protein C.

20.3 PLATELETS
Platelets are small cytoplasmic fragments, produced from megakaryocytes in the bone marrow, with a life span of 8-10 days. They are abundant in the blood, and play an important role in the arrest of bleeding:
1. Adhesion to damaged vessel walls.
2. Release of granule contents.
3. Aggregation to form a plug.
4. Provision of cofactors for clotting, with the fibrin clot that forms stabilising the platelet plug.

20.3.1 Platelet Adhesion
Following changes in the vascular endothelial lining, platelets adhere to regions of damage. This adhesion is mediated by glycoproteins on the platelet surface:
- Glycoprotein Ia – binds directly to the exposed collagen, leading to adhesion.
- Glycoprotein Ib – binds to von Willebrand factor, which then binds to subendothelial macromolecules, allowing platelet adhesion.

On adhesion to damaged vessel lining, platelets change shape. Contraction of actin and myosin filaments within platelets leads to change from smooth discs to spiny spheres with protruding pseudopodia. This change in shape is associated with exposure of glycoprotein IIb/IIIa receptors.

20.3.2 Platelet Activation and the Release Reaction
Adhesion to collagen or exposure to thrombin (allowing a positive feedback loop) leads to activation of platelets, with the release of their granule contents:
1. Collagen and thrombin activate platelet prostaglandin G_2 and H_2 synthesis from arachadonic acid.

2. These prostaglandins in turn activate the synthesis of thromboxane A$_2$, which lowers cAMP.
3. Decreases in cAMP levels increase the concentration of intracellular calcium ions, which, in turn induce the release of granules.

Platelet granules contain a number of chemical mediators, which aid in the formation of a stable clot. These include:

- ADP – induces a conformational change in the GPIIa/IIIb receptor, allowing it to bind to fibrinogen and thus localise platelet aggregation and blood clot formation to the site of injury.
- Serotonin – induces vasoconstriction.
- Thromboxane A$_2$ – induces vasoconstriction and platelet aggregation, whilst also causing more granule release. Importantly, this is the target of drugs such as aspirin, which prevent its synthesis.
- Fibrinogen – important in the formation of the fibrin clot and platelet aggregation.
- Pro-coagulant molecules e.g. platelet factor 3 – interact with the clotting cascade to accelerate the formation of a fibrin clot, which can stabilise the initial platelet plug.
- PGDF – initiates simultaneous vascular repair.

In addition to contact activation of platelets, it also appears that prostacyclin, synthesised in endothelial cells in response to damage and haemostatic mediators, is able to induce platelet degranulation.

20.3.3 Platelet Aggregation
Having adhered at the site of injury, and been activated by many factors, platelets must aggregate together to form a plug which can temporarily stop bleeding. Aggregation of platelets together forms an unstable primary haemostatic plug, which controls bleeding in the first minute or so. This plug will subsequently be stabilised by fibrin.

Various agonists, including collagen, thrombin, ADP and thromboxane A$_2$ act on receptors on the platelet surface. These induce the expression of GPIIb/IIIa receptors on the surface of the platelets. These receptors bind fibrinogen, which is present in the plasma, and thus enable the formation of links between adjacent platelets. This draws the platelets together and thus leads to aggregation. Binding of fibrinogen to these receptors induces further degranulation of the platelets, which in turn induces more GPIIb/IIIa receptor expression, and thus the process is self-perpetuating.

20.3.4 Clot Stabilisation by Fibrin
Exposure of acidic phospholipid on the outer surface of platelets activates the formation of thrombin, which in turn is able to cleave fibrinogen to fibrin (see below). Fibrin polypeptides form a meshwork with the primary platelet clot, and therefore stabilise the plug. In addition, this activates further platelets through thrombin receptors on the platelet surface.

Following the formation of the clot, it is thought calcium release within platelets, stimulated by thrombin, activates contractile proteins. This results in the retraction of the clot. In addition, as the clot evolves platelets become fused together (stimulated by ADP, thrombin and factors from the release reaction) which further stabilises the clot.

20.4 THE CLOTTING CASCADE
The clotting cascade describes the process by which fluid blood is converted into a solid gel or clot. The main event in this process is the conversion of soluble plasma fibrinogen into insoluble strands of fibrin, creating a mesh which can bind blood components (particularly platelets) together. In order

for this to occur, a sequential set of reactions happens involving 'clotting factors'. Broadly, the clotting cascade occurs in three stages:

1. Formation of prothrombin activator (factor Xa) by a chemical cascade in response to trauma.
2. Conversion of prothrombin to thrombin by factor Xa.
3. Conversion of fibrinogen to fibrin by thrombin. Fibrin enmeshes platelets, blood cells and plasma to form a stable clot.

Clotting factors (numbered I to XIII) are present in the blood as inactive precursors (zymogens) of proteolytic enzymes and cofactors. These are activated by proteolysis, with the active form being designated by the suffix 'a'. Factors XIIa, XIa, Xa, IXa and IIa (thrombin) are all serine proteases, and therefore able to cleave downstream zymogens.

Since a single active serine protease is able to cleave many zymogen molecules, the clotting cascade results in huge amplification of the initial vessel damage signal. In addition, this cascade is a good example of positive feedback, with the clot continuing to expand unless it is tightly regulated. Given the accelerating nature of the cascade, there are numerous mechanisms to slow or reverse the formation of the clot (e.g. antithrombin III, vascular endothelium heparan sulphate), thus limiting thrombus extension.

20.4.1 The Intrinsic and Extrinsic Pathways

In 1863, Joseph Lister demonstrated that blood will remain fluid if left in the excised vein of an ox, yet will clot within a few minutes if transferred to a glass vessel. It was assumed this was due to a mechanism intrinsic to the glass itself. In addition, if extrinsic tissue extracts are added to the in vitro preparation, clotting occurs within seconds. Thus, it was postulated that the initial activation of the cascade, resulting in the formation of the prothrombin activator (factor Xa) can occur by two pathways – the intrinsic and extrinsic pathways.

Extrinsic

- Activated when blood comes into contact with products of damaged tissue.
- Most important is tissue factor – an integral membrane protein released by damaged cells.
- Tissue factor activates factor VII by inducing autocatalytic cleavage in the presence of Ca^{2+} ions.
- Factor VIIa interacts with phospholipids provided by activated platelets, and converts factor X to Xa.
- This is the most important pathway for clotting *in vivo*.

Intrinsic

- Activated when blood comes into contact with a damaged surface (e.g. collagen) or artificial surface e.g. glass or catheter – factor XII adhering to a negatively charged surface.
- Involves cascade of factors XII, XI, IX and VIII.
- Results in the formation of IXa which, in conjunction with VIIIa, platelet phospholipid and Ca^{2+} ions also results in the cleavage of factor X to Xa.
- Slower response, and all necessary elements are present within the blood.
- Occurs mainly *in vitro*, with debate as to its physiological role, since factor XII deficiency has little effect on *in vivo* clotting.

In reality, there is not such a distinct separation between these two pathways. Factors from each pathway interact with the other with the final outcome being conversion of factor X to Xa.

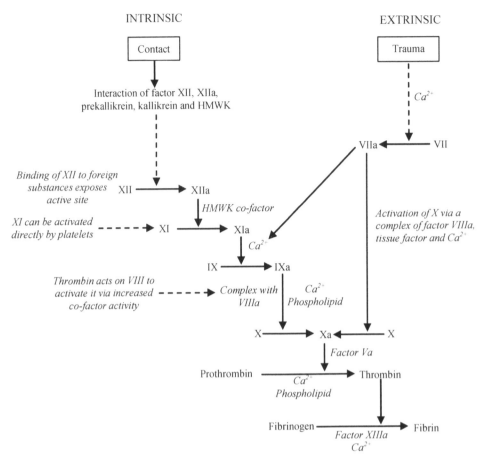

Figure 20.1 – The clotting cascade

20.4.2 Conversion of Prothrombin to Thrombin
The point of conversion of the intrinsic and extrinsic pathways is the activation of factor X to Xa. Factor Xa is known as the prothrombin activator. In the presence of Ca^{2+} ions, platelet phospholipid and factor Va, prothrombin activator cleaves prothrombin (II) to thrombin (IIa) – the main enzyme of the cascade.

20.4.3 Formation of the Fibrin Mesh
Thrombin activates soluble fibrinogen by cleavage, producing fragments which polymerise to form a fibrin meshwork. In addition, thrombin activates factor XIII in the presence of Ca^{2+}. XIIIa is a fibrinoligase and strengthens fibrin-to-fibrin links and thus further stabilises the clot.

Other roles of thrombin include:
- Platelet aggregation.
- Stimulates cell proliferation.
- Modulates smooth muscle contraction.
- Stimulate the regulatory and fibrinolytic pathway.

20.5 REGULATION
Once a clot has started to develop, it will normally extend within minutes into the surrounding blood. The self-perpetuating positive feedback nature of the cascade means that, without external factors

196

opposing its growth, a thrombus will expand until all factors have been exhausted. As such, regulation is achieved by three processes:
1. Dilution
2. Clotting inhibitors
3. Fibrinolysis

20.5.1 Dilution
Blood flow through the region of the clot means that clotting factors end up being washed away and diluted. These factors are removed by the liver and degraded by proteases.

20.5.2 Clotting Inhibitors
Clotting inhibitors act directly on factors within the cascade to inhibit their function. These include antithrombin III, protein C and protein S:
- Antithrombin III – anticoagulant secreted by regions of intact endothelium. Inhibits all the serine proteases within the cascade i.e. factors II, VII, IX, X, XI and XII. Particularly important in inactivating tissue factor-VIIa complex, and thus the extrinsic pathway.
- Protein C – activated when thrombin binds to thrombomodulin receptors in the intact epithelium. Assisted by its cofactor, protein S, it binds to factors Va and VIIa and inactivates them. This is clinically relevant since variations in factor V (e.g. in factor V Leiden) result in resistance to protein C, and thus excessive clotting.

20.5.3 Fibrinolysis
When the clotting system is activated, a set of factors that are able to dissolve away clots are also activated. These help to limit the extension of the clot beyond the region of damage, and also prevent obstruction by dissolving small clots in the circulation which may have broken off from the main area of plug formation (emboli).

The main factor in the dissolution of clots is plasmin, which is activated from plasminogen. Plasminogen is itself deposited on the fibrin strands within a thrombus, and therefore the fibrinolytic action is targeted to the area of clotting. Various factors can set off plasminogen activation including:
- Tissue plasminogen activator (tPA)
- Urokinase-type plasminogen activator (uPA)
- Kallikrein (involved in the intrinsic clotting pathway)
- Neutrophil elastase

The plasminogen activators listed above are themselves activated by the products of the clotting pathway, in particular thrombin (which has a profound effect on tPA) and other activated clotting factors.

Plasmin is an enzyme with trypsin-like activity. It digests fibrin, in addition to fibrinogen, factors II, V and VIII. Digestion of the clot results in the formation of fibrin degradation products (FDPs), some of which act as competitive inhibitors of thrombin and fibrin polymerisation. Thus, this accentuates the anti-thrombotic effects of plasmin.

Plasmin itself must be inactivated to prevent digestion of other body proteins, and thus inhibitors such as PAI-1 are present to avoid widespread damage

20.6 CLINICAL CONSIDERATIONS
Derangements in the clotting pathway can have serious implications for patients. These include excessive clotting leading to blockage of blood vessels, or problems in the cascade resulting in

thrombophilias. In addition, there are a number of medications that aim to target various areas of the clotting cascade to alter haemostasis *in vivo*.

20.6.1 Assessing Clotting
Various laboratory tests are available which test different aspects of the clotting cascade. These are useful in identifying the cause of clotting derangements e.g. haemophilia, and thus targeting treatment for these patients.

APTT (activated partial thromboplastin time)
- An activator e.g. kaolin is used to initiate contact activation.
- Reflects the function of the intrinsic pathway.
- Prolonged in factor XII, IX, VIII, X, V, II or fibrinogen deficiency e.g. haemophilia, disseminated intravascular coagulation, liver disease, heparin therapy

PT (prothrombin time)
- Tissue factor is provided.
- Tests the extrinsic pathway.
- Prolonged in factor VII, X, V, II and fibrinogen deficiency e.g. liver disease, warfarin therapy, disseminated intravascular coagulation.

TT (thrombin time):
- Exogenous thrombin added to patient plasma and time taken to clot measured.
- Prolonged if fibrinogen low, raised fibrin degradation products (D-dimers) or heparin present e.g. disseminated intravascular coagulation, heparin therapy.

20.6.2 The Importance of Vitamin K
Vitamin K is a fat-soluble vitamin that plays a vital role in the synthesis of serine proteases. In the clotting cascade, it is essential for the production of factors II, VII, IX and X. Vitamin K acts as a co-factor in the post-translation γ-carboxylation of glutamic acid residues in these factors. γ-carboxylation is essential for these factors since it allows their interaction with Ca^{2+} and negatively charged phospholipids.

Deficiency in vitamin K (e.g. due to impaired fat absorption) can therefore lead to bleeding. Low vitamin K levels in neonates can lead to haemorrhagic disease of the newborn. Thus, babies receive an intramuscular injection of the vitamin at birth.

The role of vitamin K can be exploited in the clinical setting. Warfarin antagonises vitamin K action and thus lowers clotting factor levels, preventing inappropriate clotting. Warfarin has a very narrow therapeutic range and many drug interactions, and thus administration must be carefully controlled.

20.6.3 Disorders of Bleeding
There are many diseases which affect the blood clotting cascade. These may result in an increased or decreased tendency to form clots, and can be inherited or acquired.

Inherited haemophilias
- These are usually very rare, but study of these disorders enabled coagulation cascade to be elucidated.
- Haemophilia A – X-linked recessive deficiency in Factor VIII affecting ~ 1/5000 males. Severity varies depending on the level of factor VIII in the blood. Symptoms include prolonged bleeding following accidental injury, repeated and often spontaneous bleeding

into joints and muscles. Cerebral haemorrhage is very uncommon but commonest cause of death. Can be treated with exogenous factor VIII.
- Haemophilia B – similar to haemophilia A, but caused by factor IX deficiency. This is a very rare disease.

Liver disease
- Hepatitis, cirrhosis and other liver damage may cause the clotting system to become severely depressed so that patient starts to bleed.
- This is due to insufficient synthesis of clotting factors and deficient vitamin K absorption due to decreased bile synthesis.

DIC (disseminated intravascular coagulation)
- Inappropriate and excessive activation of the haemostatic system leading to consumption of coagulation factors and platelets, and thus paradoxical bleeding.
- Characterised by low fibrinogen and high D-dimer (fibrinolytic product) level.
- May be caused by infection, shock, obstetric disorders, malignancy, burns, trauma and snake venom.

Inherited thrombophilias
- Characterised by an excessive tendency to clot.
- Examples include factor V Leiden (resistance to protein C), antithrombin III deficiency, protein C and protein S deficiencies.
- Important to identify women with factor V Leiden before administered the oral contra-ceptive pill, since these two factors combined can increase the chance of formation of deep vein thromboses.

Arterial clots
- Caused predominantly by an abnormal vessel wall.
- Platelet aggregation and clotting cascade stimulated leading to restriction in blood flow and potentially MI or stroke.
- Associated with the formation of fatty plaques and atherosclerosis.

Venous clots
- Blood clotting occurs in vessels where there has been venous stasis.
- Majority occur in deep veins of leg but liable to embolise to other areas.
- Risk factors include previous venous thromboemobolism, malignancy, immobility, surgery, travel, oral contraceptive pill, pregnancy, family history, and thrombophilia
- Typically presents as deep vein thrombosis in leg (red, swollen, warm, painful) and/or pulmonary embolus (dyspnoea, tachypnoea, pleuritic chest pain, tachycardia, cough and haemoptysis).
- Diagnosed via Doppler ultrasound, D-dimer and CT pulmonary angiogram.
- Treat with low molecular weight heparin and warfarin.
- Can be prevented by stopping the pill 4 weeks before operations and early mobilisation after operations, along with heparin and support stockings.

20.6.4 Drugs Affecting Clotting
There are many medications that can be used to either increase or decrease a patient's tendency to clot. In addition, it is possible to destroy pre-existing clots.

Anticoagulants
- Heparin – heparin or low-molecular weight heparin are injectable anticoagulants. They stabilise the association between antithrombin III and factors Xa and II, thus increasing its anticoagulant effect. Dosing with LMWH is much easier to control, and thus it is preferred.
- Warfarin – oral anticoagulant that inhibits the reduction of vitamin K. As such, warfarin inhibits the synthesis of factors II, VII, IX and X. The effect of warfarin is monitored closely with the patient's INR (international normalised ratio) which gives and indication of the coagulability of the blood.
- Antithrombin III-independent anticoagulants – hirudin and argatroban, which are direct inhibitors of thrombin function.

Antiplatelet drugs
- Aspirin – inhibits cyclooxygenase irreversibly, thus preventing the synthesis of thromboxane A_2 by platelets and therefore aggregation. Also inhibits vascular endothelium prostaglandin I_2 synthesis (an aggregation inhibitor), but endothelial cells are able to synthesise new cyclooxygenase, unlike platelets, thus tipping the balance towards prevention of clotting.
- Clopidogrel – inhibits platelet aggregation response to ADP.
- GPIIb/IIIa antagonists – examples include abciximab and tirofiban. Inhibit multiple pathways of platelet activation, which converge on GPIIb/IIIa receptors.
- Others – dipyridamole (phosphodiesterase inhibitor) and epoprostenol (synthetic prostaglandin I_2).

Fibrinolytic agents
- Streptokinase – activates plasminogen and thus fibrinolysis. Used to prevent mortality in acute MI (but must be administered within 12 hours). Isolated from streptococci bacteria, and therefore its action is blocked by anti-streptococcal antibodies.
- Tissue plasminogen activators (tPA) – recombinant forms of human tPA, such as alteplase and duteplase. Not affected by anti-streptococcal antibodies.

Pro-thrombotic agents
- Recombinant factor VIII and IX in patients with haemophilia.
- Tranexamic acid – anti-fibrinolytic agent, used in haemorrhage associated with fibrinolytic agents.
- Vitamin K – prevention of haemolytic disease of the newborn, liver disease-associated bleeding and treatment of warfarin overdose.

CHAPTER 21

Antibodies and Complement

21.1 ANTIBODIES: IMMUNOGLOBULINS

21.1.1 The Immune System
The immune system serves a vital role in the recognition and destruction of potentially pathogenic organisms (bacteria, fungi, protozoa and viruses). In addition, the immune system is able to recognise damaged or altered host cells, and facilitate their removal. Broadly speaking, the immune system is divided into innate and acquired systems.

21.1.1.1 Innate Immunity
The innate immune system is described as being non-specific, since it does not require the production of molecules or responses specific to an invading organism. There are three main elements to the innate immune system:

Anatomical
- Skin – provides a physical barrier, and has acidic pH which prevents microbial growth.
- Mucous membranes – also provide physical barrier, and have mucous covered and ciliated surfaces to entrap and expel foreign organisms.
- Commensal organisms – colonies of bacteria normally present throughout the body, which do not cause disease in healthy individuals. These compete with pathogenic organisms (e.g. for nutrients, receptor binding sites) and thus prevent them from reproducing.

Physiological
- Inflammation – series of cellular and molecular interactions, leading to activation of immune cells, the generation of a fever, 'leakiness' of capillaries and increased regenerative processes.
- High temperature of fever (as part of inflammation), allowing pathogen protein denaturation.
- Acidic pH of the stomach.
- Complement system – destroys micro-organisms, facilitates phagocytosis, interacts with antibodies etc.

Phagocytic
- Phagocytes (monocytes, neutrophils, macrophages) which recognise shared molecular patterns (pathogen associated patterns) present in many pathogens, and subsequently engulf and digest micro-organisms.
- Activated phagocytes also release many cytokines, activating innate responses such as fever, and also stimulating acquired immune responses.

This is a very brief overview of the innate immune system, and it shall not be discussed in further detail.

21.1.1.2 Acquired Immunity
The acquired immune system leads to responses that are specific to each microorganism. The core requirement of the acquired immune system is to recognise particular antigens (molecules which lead to the generation of an antibody) and launch a cellular and humoral response to that antigen. Antigens are present on the surface of microorganisms, and therefore recognition of an antigen by the acquired immune system leads to a response against that microorganism.

The acquired immune system must fulfil four main criteria:

1. Be specific for antigens.
2. Be diverse, allowing the recognition of multiple antigens.
3. Have a system for immunological memory – 'remembering' when an antigen has been seen before, and generating a stronger response to it on second exposure.
4. Distinguish between self and non-self antigens, preventing autoimmune disease.

The acquired immune system relies on white blood cells known as lymphocytes, which originate from stem cell precursors in the bone marrow. These are broadly divided into T and B-lymphocytes, which make up the cellular and humoral parts respectively of the acquired immune system:

Cellular response
- Mediated by T-lymphocytes.
- Responses to microorganisms possessing a particular antigen are carried out by the cells themselves.
- Destruction of microorganisms is performed by cytotoxic T-lymphocytes (killer cells) with help from helper T-lymphocytes.

Humoral response
- Mediated by antibodies, generated by activated B-lymphocytes (plasma cells) specific for a particular antigen.
- Antibodies bind to the surface of microorganisms, and then interact with other immune cells (see below), inducing a response.
- Destruction is not preformed by the B-lymphocytes or antibodies themselves, but other cells.

In order for the acquired immune system to respond correctly to invading microorganisms, there is communication with the innate immune system. This involves the production of molecular signals produced by phagocytes on engulfing foreign organisms, and the 'presentation' of epitopes (immunologically active regions of an antigen, which actually bind to the antibody) to B and T-lymphocytes by these phagocytes.

21.1.2 Antibodies
Antibodies (also known as immunoglobulins) are soluble proteins, produced by activated B-lymphocytes (plasma cells). They have a unique structure which enables them to be specific to particular antigens, whilst simultaneously inducing downstream effects.

21.1.2.1 Antibody Production
The humoral immune system is able to recognise a huge number of antigens, present on a multitude of different organisms. However, when a particular pathogen invades the body, only some of these antibodies will be specific for antigens on that pathogen. Thus, to make the response as efficient as possible, the body must select the B-lymphocytes capable of producing only antibodies particular for that pathogen, and then allow that B-lymphocyte to replicate and secrete large amounts of specific antibody. The way in which this happens is described by the clonal selection theory:

1. Before an animal even encounters a foreign antigen, it possesses a huge repertoire of B-lymphocytes, each of which is capable of producing one specific antibody. This antibody is anchored in the cell membrane of that B-lymphocyte, allowing it to act as a receptor for external antigens. However, there are only one or two B-lymphocytes with each specific antibody – insufficient for production of sufficient levels of antibody to protect against invading pathogens.

2. A foreign antigen is encountered, and displayed to many B-lymphocytes.

3. The B-lymphocyte with surface antibody that binds strongly to the antigen is activated.

4. Activation of this B-lymphocyte leads to generation of clones – rapid multiplication of B-lymphocytes, each with identical antigen specificity.

5. These lymphocytes mature into short lived plasma cells, with the capacity to secrete huge amounts (2000 molecules per second) of specific antibody, which may now bind to the antigen on the surface of the invading pathogen.

6. Long-lived memory B-lymphocytes are generated. These express the same membrane-bound antibody as the activated B-lymphocytes, but are able to transform into plasma cells and multiply much more rapidly. Thus, if the particular antigen is encountered again, the second response is faster and greater (immunological memory).

In order to maximise exposure to antigens and the efficient generation of a response, the body possesses lymphoid tissue. Lymphoid tissue is structurally designed such that antigens may be brought by phagocytes, and presented to a multitude of lymphocytes allowing for clonal selection. In addition, when a specific lymphocyte has been selected, multiplication of these lymphocytes and the production of antibodies by plasma cells also occurs within lymphoid tissue. Types of lymphoid tissue include:
- Mucosa-associated lymphoid tissue – lymphoid tissue present at the mucosal surfaces (e.g. in the tonsils, GI tract, respiratory tract, genito-urinary tract) close to the luminal surface, such that antigens within the lumen may be delivered rapidly and a response generated close to portals of pathogen entry.
- Lymph nodes – drain lymph from around the body, and often present in collections e.g. cervical chains in the neck.
- Spleen – the spleen has a profuse blood supply, allowing contact of cells within lymphoid tissue with antigens that may be present in the blood.

In addition to lymphoid tissue, plasma cells and antibody production are focussed in breast tissue (for secretion of antibodies in breast milk) and the bone marrow (since B-lymphocytes mature in the marrow).

21.1.2.2 Antibody Structure
There are five different classes of antibody. Each of these has a slightly different structure. However, the archetypal antibody, used to describe the general structure of antibodies is immunoglobulin G (IgG).

IgG is a Y-shaped molecule, consisting of four polypeptide chains joined together by disulphide bonds. There are two light chains (around 220 amino acids in length) and two heavy chains (440 amino acids in length). The antibody possesses variable and constant regions, different domains and two distinct fragments (antigen binding and crystallising fragments).

Variable and constant regions
- Comparison of amino acid sequences of various immunoglobulins has demonstrated that the N-terminal region of each light and heavy chain is highly variable.
- In addition, the C-terminal region of each light and heavy chain is constant.

- The N-terminal sequences of the light and heavy chains form the antigen-binding region of the antibody, hence they are highly variable to allow different antigen specificities.
- Further analysis has demonstrated three 'hypervariable' regions in the N-terminal sequences of each chain. Three-dimensional studies have demonstrated these hypervariable regions are concentrated in the antigen-binding regions of the N-terminals.

Antibody domains
- Each light chain consists of two three-dimensional domains, each of around 110 amino acids. These represent the constant and variable regions of the light chain.
- Similarly, the heavy chains are divided into 110 amino acid domains. There is one variable domain, and three repeating constant unit domains.

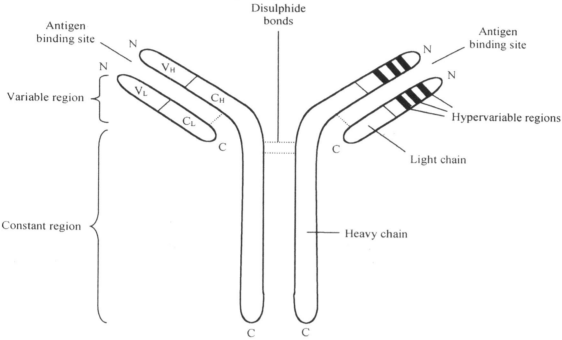

Figure 21.1 – Antibody structure

Antibody fragments
- It is possible to digest antibodies into their constituent parts using enzymes.
- Papain is a protease which acts on the heavy chains – digestion by this enzyme generates three fragments. One consisting solely of the constant regions of heavy chains, and two consisting of both constant and variable regions of heavy and light chains, connected by disulphide bonds.
- It has been demonstrated that the fragment consisting only of heavy chains possesses no antigen-binding capacity. However, it is able to stimulate other cells by interactions with receptors on their surface. Thus, this is shown to be the 'effector' portion of the antibody, and is known as the Fc region, since it readily crystallises.
- Similarly, the released arms of the antibody, consisting of variable and constant regions have been demonstrated to have antigen binding ability, but are not able to stimulate effector responses. These are therefore known as the antigen-binding fragments (Fab).
- In contrast to papain, pepsin can be used to digest the antibody lower down the heavy chain. Thus, the connections between the two arms are maintained, demonstrating the role of the two arms in cross-linking antigens when binding simultaneously.

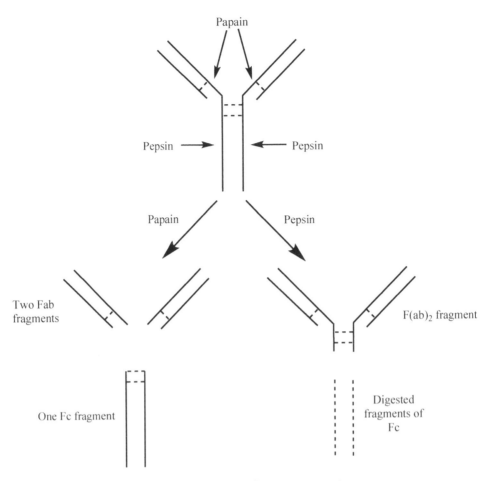

Figure 21.2 – Antibody digestion experiments

21.1.2.3 Classes of Antibody

Humans have five different classes of antibody, each of which differs in structure and function. These are classified according to their heavy chain constant regions, each of which is called an isotype. The five classes are:

- IgA – possesses α heavy chains. There are two subclasses of IgA.
- IgD – possesses δ heavy chains.
- IgE – possesses ε heavy chains.
- IgG – possesses γ heavy chains. There are four subclasses of IgG, each with slightly different γ chains.
- IgM – possesses μ heavy chains.

In addition, an antibody may possess either a κ or λ light chain, but never both together. The functional significance of this is not known.

IgM

- Exists as a pentamer in combination with another polypeptide – the J-chain – which initiates polymerisation.

- Has 10 binding sites, and can therefore bind very tightly to pathogens with multiple copies of the same antigen on their surface.
- Binding induces changes in the Fc region, leading to complement activation and pathogen destruction.
- Activates phagocytosis by macrophages (opsonisation).
- Present in some secretions, and can be used as a B-lymphocyte receptor when present in the cell membrane.
- Given its multiple binding capacity, this is the first antibody produced in response to a new antigen.
- Short half life of 5 days.

IgG

- Main immunoglobulin in the bloodstream late in the initial response to a pathogen (as IgM decreases) or in response to second exposure to an antigen (i.e. the memory response).
- Can activate complement and opsonise much like IgM.
- Only antibody able to cross the placenta, providing protection to the foetus and newborn child. However, turnover means that once maternal antibody has been depleted (after around two months) the newborn is susceptible to infection until their immune system matures.
- Some suggestion it appears in mothers milk, and therefore provides protection to the newborn child.
- Has the longest half life, at 23 days in the serum.

IgA

- Exists as a dimer, also being joined by a J-region.
- Has 4 binding sites.
- Main class of secreted antibody, being present in the tears, saliva, lungs, intestine and breast milk.
- Very important in defence against pathogens at mucosal surfaces.
- Half life of 6 days in the serum.

IgE

- Cross-linking antibody, which binds to receptors on the surface of mast cells.
- Induces degranulation of mast cells, and subsequently the release of histamine, leukotrienes and various other cytokines.
- Mast cell signals activate eosinophils, which are important in the protection against parasites.
- Also lead to allergic responses when activated by non-pathogenic antigens.
- Mast cell signals induce vasodilation and increased vascular permeability, leading to symptoms such as those seen in asthma and hay fever.
- May induce death through shock in extreme situations (e.g. peanut allergies).
- Half life of 2.5 days in the serum.

IgD

- Found on the surface of mature B-lymphocytes, and acts as the B-cell receptor.
- Some is found in secretions, but the function of this is unclear.
- Short half life of only 3 days in the serum.

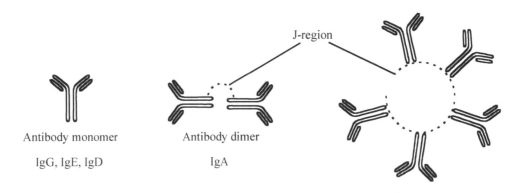

Figure 21.3 – Antibody classes

	IgG	IgA	IgM	IgE	IgD
Molecular weight	150000	150000-600000	900000	190000	150000
Normal serum level (g/L)	6-13	0.8-3	0.4-2.5	0.0003	0.03
Form	Monomer	Dimer	Pentamer	Monomer	Monomer
Binding sites	2	4	10	2	2
Serum half-life (days)	23	6	5	2.5	3
Complement activation	Yes	No	Yes	No	No
Crosses placenta	Yes	No	No	No	No
B-cell receptor	No	No	Yes	No	Yes
Opsonisation	Yes	No	Yes	No	No
Secreted	No	Yes	Yes	No	No
Mast cell degranulation	No	No	No	Yes	No

21.1.2.4 Antibody Function

Antibodies act as the effector arm of the humoral immune response. They are able to bind specifically to antigens, and induce downstream effects using their constant regions. Broadly, the roles of antibodies are:

- Agglutination – cross linking of bound antigen, particularly on the surface of viruses and bacteria, forming clusters which immobilise the organism and make them a target for phagocytosis.
- Opsonisation – coating of antigen, and activation of phagocytes to engulf the organism through Fc receptors on the phagocyte. This also activates the phagocyte to produce signalling molecules.
- Mucous membranes – binding to antigens on pathogen surfaces to prevent their entry into the body.
- Activation of complement – antigen-antibody complexes are able to activate the complement pathway, and thus induce cell lysis and inflammatory responses.
- Neutralisation – bind to antigens such as bacterial toxin, preventing them from having their effects e.g. tetanus toxin neutralised by exogenous IgG injection.
- Receptors for B-lymphocytes.

The variable regions of the antibody are responsible for antigen binding. 15-20% of the variable region consists of the hypervariable sections (also known as complementarity-determining regions - CDRs), and these are responsible for the actual binding to the antigen. In order for antibodies to operate appropriately, 4 of the 6 CDRs must bind with epitopes on the antigen. Interactions between the antigen and antibody are based on non-covalent forces (i.e. ionic, hydrogen and van der Waals forces) which are relatively weak on their own. Thus, at least four CDRs must be bound in order to stabilise contact and induce changes in the Fc region.

The strength of interaction between antigen and antibody is determined by the affinity and avidity of the antibody:
- Affinity – strength of interaction between a single antigen-binding site and single epitope. Low affinity antibodies can bind only weakly, whilst high affinity antibodies bind strongly and are less likely to dissociate from the antigen.
- Avidity – describes the strength of multiple interactions between a multivalent antibody and an antigen. Much better measure of an antibody's binding capacity in vivo, and is used to compensate for low affinity (e.g. IgM). Cooperative binding also occurs, with the binding of one CDR leading to an increased probability of binding at a second site.

The constant regions of an antibody determine its biological effector function. Since many of the functions of antibodies are shared, regardless of their antigen specificity, the Fc region varies little between antibodies of the same class. However, constant region variation between classes allows different effector functions:
- Mast cell interaction – IgE Fc regions are specifically designed to bind to receptors on mast cells and induce degranulation.
- Macrophage and neutrophils interaction – IgG and IgM Fc regions are designed to interact with Fc receptors on phagocytes and induce opsonisation and activation, whilst also triggering the complement pathway.
- Secretion – IgG and IgA have particularly hydrophilic Fc regions, allowing movement across the placenta and secretion into tears, colostrum and the gut respectively.
- Membrane binding – IgD has a particularly hydrophobic Fc region, allowing implantation into the membrane.

Affinity maturation and class switching
- Over a period of time, a single B-lymphocyte will change the class of antibody it produces in response to external signals (predominantly interleukins).
- Class-switching allows alteration in the function of the antibodies produced, such that a serum-based IgM response may, for example, be transformed into a mucosa-based IgA response if the pathogen is concentrated at mucosal surfaces.
- Importantly, class-switching has no effect on the variable region of the antibody – the specificity for the antigen remains the same.
- Affinity maturation also occurs, in which prolonged exposure to an antigen allows subtle changes in the CDRs of the antigens being produced, such that they have a higher affinity for the antigen.

21.1.3 Clinical Considerations
21.1.3.1 Antibody Deficiencies
Given the central importance of antibodies to defence against infectious disease, it is unsurprising that deficiency can have serious consequences. There is a range of antibody disease, with some affecting only a small population of B-lymphocytes and thus having significantly less effects than those that act universally.

Antibodies are particularly important in defence against capsulated bacteria, which can resist direct phagocytosis. This includes Staphylococci, Pneumococci and Haemophilus species of bacteria. Thus, particular infections are prevalent in those with antibody deficiency:

- Respiratory tract infections (90%) – sinusitis, otitis media, bronchitis, pneumonia.
- Skin infections (20%) – abscesses.
- GI and liver infections (13%) – diarrhoea and malabsorption.
- Bone infections (6%) – osteomyelitis.
- Joint infections (6%) – infective arthritis.

Bruton's X-linked antibody deficiency
- X-linked disease, thus affecting boys.
- Defect in B-cell tyrosine kinase, preventing maturation of pre-B-cells into mature lymphocytes.
- B-lymphocytes absent from the blood and lymphoid organs.
- Very low or absent IgG, IgM and IgA in the blood.
- Poor prognosis given broad effect.

Common variable immunodeficiency disorders
- Group of conditions characterised by abnormal B-lymphocyte to T-lymphocyte interactions.
- Low levels of IgG, IgM and IgA (although variable) and can thus mimic Bruton's.
- Differentiated from Bruton's since B-cells are present in the blood, and there may be disordered T-cell function leading to associated autoimmunity, allergy and malignancy.
- Unknown pathogenesis so a diagnosis of exclusion.

Selective IgA deficiency
- Commonest antibody deficiency (1 in 700).
- Normal IgM and IgG production, but there is a lack of serum and secretory IgA due to a specific plasma cell problem.
- May be asymptomatic.

Secondary antibody deficiency
- Much commoner than primary deficiencies, and normally occur through altered production or increased loss.
- Prematurity – transient antibody deficiency, although maintained for up to 6 months.
- Antibody loss – excessive burns, renal disease and protein-losing enteropathies.
- Decreased production – B-cell malignancies, medication and infections.

Management of serious antibody deficiencies involves replacement with infusions of IgG, whilst treating with antibiotics, close monitoring for signs of infection and potential treatment of the underlying cause.

21.1.3.2 Therapeutic Antibodies
Knowledge of the ways in which antibodies operate has allowed their usage as a tool. They are a valuable resource in both clinical and experimental settings.

Immunisation of patients who are suspected of having tetanus (and thus tetanus toxin) involves the injection of a preparation of antibodies to neutralise the toxin. Similarly, antibodies have been generated that may target certain cells (e.g. tumour cells, other immune cells), either to induce their lysis and removal, or to alter their behaviour through blocking or stimulation of receptors.

The generation of monoclonal antibodies (antibodies which all have identical epitope specificity) has been made possible using specific B-lymphocytes fused with lymphocyte tumour cells, known as myeloma cells. The resulting 'hybridoma' produces a large amount of a single type of antibody. This has been used in laboratory research, since tagged antibodies can now be used to locate particular molecules or fragments on cells or in solution. This has allowed more accurate diagnosis of diseases such as cancer, with the detection of cells expressing tumour markers in tissue samples.

21.2 COMPLEMENT

The complement system forms a major effector component of the humoral immune system. It consists of over 30 soluble plasma and membrane proteins, operating in a cascade similar to that of haemostasis, resulting in particular terminal effects. Thus, the activated product of one step becomes the enzyme for the catalysis of the next step. The proteins and glycoproteins (numbered C1-C9) are synthesised mainly by the liver, but also by monocytes and tissue macrophages.

The main components of the complement pathway – C1 to C9 – circulate in the plasma in their inactive form. Activation of these components involves cleavage, removing an inhibitory fragment and generating 'a' and 'b' fragments. Both of these fragments are active, yet in general the 'a' part diffuses from the site of generation to act, whilst the 'b' fragment, which is larger, binds to targets

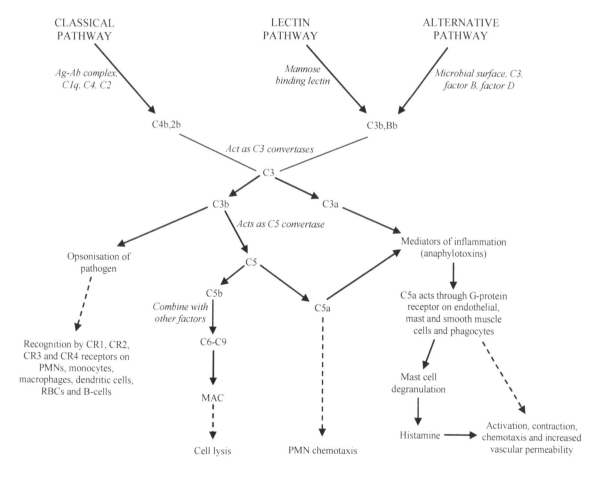

Figure 21.4 – The complement cascade

near the site of activation. In addition to acting alone, complement fragments may form functional complexes.

There are three ways of activating the complement cascade (Classical, Alternative and Lectin pathways), yet these all converge on a terminal reaction sequence, starting with the conversion of C3 to C3a and C3b. The terminal reaction sequence results in the generation of the membrane attack complex (MAC), as well as opsonins and inflammatory mediators.

21.2.1 Activation of the Complement Cascade
The complement cascade can be activated by three pathways. Each is able to distinguish pathogenic patterns, from those of the host, preventing erroneous activation:
- Classical pathway – antigen-antibody complexes.
- Alternative pathway – microbial surfaces.
- Lectin pathway – mannose-binding lectin interacting with bacteria.

21.2.1.1 Classical Pathway
The classical pathway is triggered by antigen-antibody complexes, or by the binding of antibody to antigen on a suitable target, such as a bacterial cell wall. Only IgM and IgG are able to activate the classical pathway.

The binding of antibody to antigen induces a conformational change in the Fc portion of the antibody. This exposes the binding site for C1q and thus the cascade is triggered:
1. C1q binds via C1q binding sites in the C_H2 domain of the immunoglobulin.
2. Binding of C1q activates the formation of the C1 complex (C1q with C1s and C1r).
3. C1s hydrolyses C4, generating C4a and C4b.
4. C4b attaches to the target surface, whilst C2 binds to C4b allowing C1s to cleave C2 to C2a and C2b.
5. C2a and C4b combine into a complex which acts as C3 convertase.
6. C3 convertase (C4b2a) is able to activate C3 to C3a and C3b – the reaction shared with the other pathways of activation.

In order to be activated, each C1q molecule must bind at least two Fc sites on an antibody. When pentameric IgM binds to an antigen, three sites for C1q binding are exposed, and thus IgM pentamers can activate complement alone. IgG, however, has only one C1q binding site exposed. Thus, additional IgG-antigen complexes are required to activate the complement pathway.

21.2.1.2 Alternative Pathway
The alternative pathway is initiated by cell-surface components which are foreign to the host. In particular, bacterial cell wall constituents may activate complement this way. The alternative pathways involves four serum proteins:
- C3
- Factor B
- Factor D
- Properdin

Under normal conditions, a small amount of C3 is spontaneously hydrolysed, generating C3a and C3b. C3b binds to both host and bacterial cells. However, host cells have membrane bound enzymes which inactivate C3b, preventing complement activation. Bacterial cells do not have this property:
1. C3b binds to bacterial cell surface and remains active.

2. C3b is bound by factor B.
3. Factor B is cleaved by factor D, releasing a small fragment (Ba) and thus generating C3bBb complex.
4. C3bBb has the same C3 convertase activity as C4b2a, thus generating C3a and C3b.
5. The C3b generated may then bind again to the bacterial surface, leading to a positive-feedback loop.

21.2.1.3 Lectin Pathway
The lectin pathway is activated by serum protein mannose-binding lectin interacting with mannose in bacterial cell walls. This complex leads to the generation of C3bBb and thus the activation of C3. Importantly, mannose is not present in mammalian cell membranes.

21.2.1.4 Amplification and Control
The complement cascade is subject to amplification. Since each activated component may catalyse the next step in the cascade many times, a small initial signal is amplified resulting in a larger final effect. For example, one molecule of C3 convertase may generate over 200 molecules of C3b, leading to signal amplification at this stage of the pathway.

Given the amplification potential of the complement cascade, regulation is particularly important. In addition, there is the possibility of activation on the surface of host cells. As such, complement components are extremely labile, and spontaneously inactivate when they diffuse away from target cells. In addition, there are a series of regulatory proteins, present on the surface of host cells and within the plasma. These include:
- C1 inhibitor – binds C1r and C1s, preventing C4 and C2 activation.
- Complement receptor 1 – inactivates C3b and C4b.
- Decay-accelerating factor – inactivates C3b and C4b.
- CD59 – prevents C5b, C6 and C7 complex binding to the membrane.
- C4b-binding protein – binds to C4b, displacing C2b.

21.2.2 Roles of the Complement Cascade
The pathways of complement activation converge on the generation of C3a and C3b. These two fragments subsequently initiate the effector cascade of the complement pathway. There are three broad effector arms of the complement cascade:
- Opsonisation
- MAC formation
- Inflammation and neutrophils chemotaxis

Effect	Component
Cell lysis	C5b-C9 (MAC)
Inflammation:	
Mast cell and basophil degranulation	C3a, C4a, C5a
Leukocyte chemotaxis	C3a, C5a
Platelet aggregation	C3a, C5a
Hydrolytic enzyme release from neutrophils	C5a
Opsonisation	C3b, C4b
Viral neutralisation	C3b, MAC

C3a Pathways

The main role of C3a is to act as an anaphylatoxin. Thus, it is able to initiate inflammation, resulting in the degranulation of mast cells and basophils, attraction of leukocytes, aggregation of platelets and release of hydrolytic enzymes from neutrophils.

Initiation is an essential part of the initial response to pathogens, and feeds into the adaptive immune system, stimulating a specific antibody and cell-dependent response.

C3b Pathways

C3b may act as an opsonin. Thus, it coats immune complexes and particular antigens to make phagocytosis easier. C3b interacts with CR1, CR2, CR3 and CR4 receptors on the surface of phagocytes (neutrophils, monocytes, macrophages, dendritic cells) as well as red blood cells and B-lymphocytes stimulating downstream effector responses.

In addition, C3b binds to C4b2b or C3bBb (C3 convertase) complex, forming the C5 convertase. This enzyme complex leads to the generation of C5a and C5b. C5a works in much the same way as C3a, initiating inflammation and neutrophils chemotaxis. C5b, however, is important in the formation of the membrane attack complex.

C5b binds to the surface of bacteria, and attracts components C6, C7, C8 and C9. Together, these form the MAC, which displaces membrane phospholipids, forming a transmembrane channel within the bacterium. This channel allows the free movement of ions and small molecules and thus the influx of water and loss of electrolytes from the bacterial cytoplasm. This results in lysis of the bacterial cell.

21.2.3 Clinical Considerations

As with antibodies, deficiency or problems with components of the complement cascade can compromise a patient's ability to deal with infections. In addition, failure of regulation can result in excessive responses to innocuous stimuli. Examples include:

- C1, 4, 2 and 3 deficiency – results in an immune complex disease similar to systemic lupus erythematosus.
- C3, H, 1 and 5 deficiency – repeated and serious pyogenic bacterial infections.
- C5-9 deficiency – particular susceptibility to Neisseria infection (meningitis and gonorrhoea).
- C1q inhibitor deficiency – angioedema due to excessive kinin release e.g. massive lip swelling after trauma.

214

Index

218

Lightning Source UK Ltd.
Milton Keynes UK
UKOW06f1841101114

241416UK00011B/636/P